Family Health 2024

Elevate Your Health Game, Thrive Together, and Unleash the

Power of Well-Being!

By

Jocelyn J. Barker

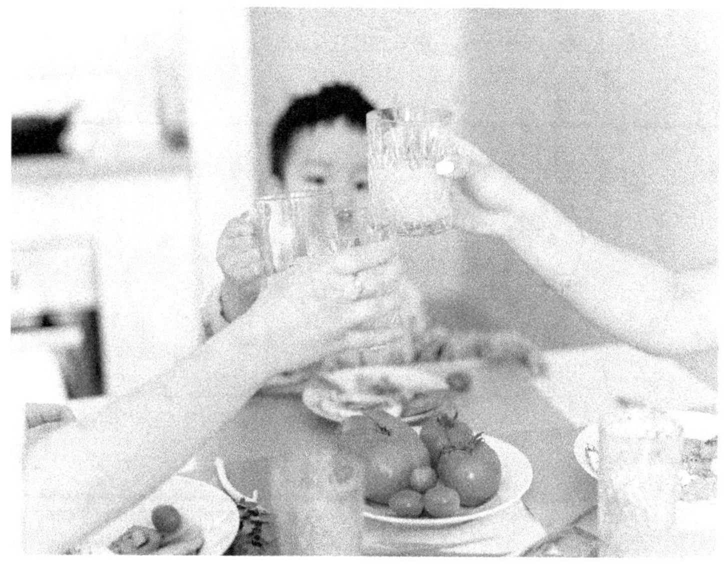

Healthy Family Lifestyles exposed

Copyright

Jocelyn J. Barker's 2023. All intellectual property rights are reserved. Except for brief quotations included in critical reviews and certain other noncommercial uses permitted by copyright law, no part of this publication may be reproduced, distributed, or transmitted in any structure or using any and all means, including copying, recording, or other electronic or mechanical techniques, without the publisher's earlier composed consent.

Disclaimer

The content in this book is provided solely for general informative purposes. It is not meant to provide medical, legal, or other professional advice. Readers are recommended to seek particular counsel tailored to their situation from relevant professionals. The author and publisher make no representations or warranties about the truth, applicability, fitness, or completeness of this book's contents. They provide no express or implied warranties about merchantability or suitability for a particular purpose. In no event shall the author or publisher be held accountable for any loss or Other damages may include, but are not limited to, special, incidental, consequential, or other damages. As usual, seek the advice of a qualified specialist. Third-party product, rate, or website references are subject to change without notice. The author and publisher do not guarantee the correctness of the content of such information and are not liable for any errors or omissions.

ABOUT THE AUTHOR

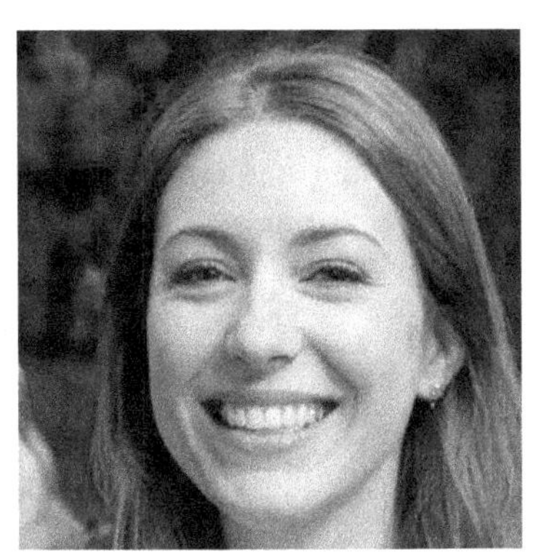

Meet Jocelyn J. Barker, the driving force behind "Family Health 2024." Jocelyn J. Barker is not just an author but a passionate advocate for family health and healthy living. With a heart dedicated to nurturing the well-being of families, she brings a wealth of knowledge and a personal touch to the pages of this book.

Jocelyn J. Barker] believes in the transformative power of small, intentional actions in shaping a family's health journey. Her expertise in family health is not just derived from textbooks but from the day-to-day experiences and triumphs of real families navigating the maze of modern living.

Having spent years immersed in the world of health and wellness, [Jocelyn J. Barker understands that well-being is not a one-size-fits-all concept. Through her writing, she aims to inspire and guide families toward a path of joyous living, where health becomes an integral and enjoyable part of their story.

Beyond the pages of this book, Jocelyn J. Barker continues to explore new avenues of promoting family health. Whether through community initiatives, speaking engagements, or her online presence, she remains committed to empowering families to thrive physically, mentally, and emotionally.

So, as you embark on the journey laid out in "Family Health 2024," know that you are in the hands of an author who not only talks the talk but walks the walk when it comes to building a healthier and happier family life. Here's to Jocelyn J. Barker and her dedication to the well-being of families everywhere!

Table of Content

INTRODUCTION

Step into the lively universe of "Family Wellbeing 2024: Raise Your Wellbeing Game, Flourish Together, and Release the Force of Prosperity!" "This isn't just a book; it's your guide to a better, more joyful day in the unique setting of 2024."

In the pages that follow, we'll explore the steadily developing territory of family prosperity, offering a new point of view on the convergence of wellbeing, satisfaction, and strength. As the world speeds up, so does the requirement for an all encompassing way to deal with health, and this guide is your complete tool stash for developing imperativeness inside your nuclear family.

From the actual underpinning of wellbeing to the powerful combination of wellness schedules reasonable for all ages, every part is a stepping stone towards a better, more associated family. Plunge into the subtleties of careful nourishment, investigate the complexities of rest concordance, and disentangle the sorcery of mental health as we dive into pressure busting systems intended for the whole family.

This book is a compass, directing you through the mind boggling scene of family wellbeing and offering bits of knowledge, methodologies, and functional tips to raise your family's essentialness. From laying out a strong starting point for wellbeing to investigating the domains of wellness combination, careful sustenance, and the wizardry of mental health, every section is made to reverberate with the different necessities of your relatives.

This isn't just about endorsing schedules; embracing a way of life cultivates aggregate prosperity. Find how elective treatments consistently coordinate into your day to day life, investigate the most recent in tech devices for wellbeing, and set out on family undertakings that bond as well as lift imperativeness.

Along these lines, affix your safety belts, open your psyches to additional opportunities, and go along with us in this groundbreaking excursion. " Family

Wellbeing 2024" isn't simply an aid — it's a challenge to flourish together, opening the maximum capacity of your family's prosperity in the thrilling scene of the present and the promising future ahead.

Embracing a Wellness Revolution

Venturing into the section on "Embracing a Wellness Revolution" wants to make a way for another period for your family in the pages of "Family Wellbeing 2024." Envision it as a new beginning, an opportunity to rework the tale of your family's well-being in a world humming with energizing prospects.

This piece of the excursion isn't just about wellness schedules or diet plans; it's an entire mindset shift. It's like choosing to move to another beat — a beat that reverberates with the congruity of body, psyche, and soul. We're discussing an unrest that goes past the typical wellbeing exhortation, pushing you to reevaluate how you approach life's promising and less promising times.

Picture this: your family, furnished with a healthy outlook, exploring pressure, praising triumphs, and fashioning more grounded associations. It's not just about arriving at a wellbeing objective; about making a way of life upholds your family's novel beat.

Envision strolling into the "Embracing a Wellbeing Transformation" section of "Family Wellbeing 2024" as though you're going into a room loaded up with the fragrance of new conceivable outcomes. It's not only a section; it's an encouragement to reconsider how your family approaches wellbeing, a call to embrace a health transformation that is both individual and group.

This isn't tied in with keeping a bunch of guidelines; about taking on a mentality changes the manner in which you view prosperity. It's like choosing to paint on a more extensive material, consolidating actual wellbeing as well as mental and profound health. Consider it an upset that welcomes your family to move to its interesting musicality of wellbeing.

Here, we're not simply talking about diets and activities; we're exploring how your family's approach to well-being can be a dynamic, developing story. It's tied in with implanting day to day decisions with a goal, understanding that every little choice adds to the bigger embroidered artwork of your family's well being.

As we explore this upheaval together, expect accounts that vibe interesting, tips that are reasonable, and bits of knowledge that flash those "aha" minutes. Consider this section as an aide, tenderly reassuring you to step into a way of life that upholds your family's prosperity process, for the time being as well as for the long stretch.

In this way, here's to embracing a wellbeing upheaval — an excursion where wellbeing is definitely not an unbending objective, however a dynamic, continuous investigation for your family in the dazzling scene of 2024 and beyond. We should make well-being a no nonsense piece of your family's story, where every day unfurls another page in this energizing, wellbeing centered narrative.

As we plunge into this revolution, anticipate genuine stories, pragmatic tips, and a ton of motivation. Consider it a guide, directing you through a shift that is a one-time thing as well as a consistent excursion. Thus, here's to embracing a wellbeing revolution — where wellbeing isn't an objective; it's an energetic, continuous story for your family in the thrilling scene of 2024 and beyond.

Welcome to a chapter that's all about making well-being a living, breathing part of your family's day to day existence.

The Journey to Family Well-being

Entering "The Journey to Family Well-being" in "Family Health 2024" means stepping onto a path that has been cleaned of powerful energies and meaningful associations. This section is definitely not a bunch of rules; think about it more like a well disposed guide, sharing stories and bits of knowledge to assist your family with exploring the exciting bends in the road toward a better, more joyful life.

Envision this excursion as an excursion where you find the panoramic detours of prosperity together. It's not necessary to focus on arriving at a particular spot however, taking in the scenery, relishing each insight en route. We're looking at making an energy where wellbeing turns into a characteristic piece of your family's story, not a task but rather a common experience.

As we roll through this part, we'll explore the significance of open communication inside the family. It's tied in with making a space where everybody feels appreciated, comprehended, and upheld. We'll address putting forth objectives together and understanding how every individual's wellbeing resembles an interconnecting piece that finishes the master plan of family strength.

You'll track down bits of knowledge on meshing solid schedules and ceremonies into your regular routine, making wellbeing a consistent piece of your family's musicality. There's no need to focus on severe guidelines yet finding what works for your remarkable group.

In this way, here's to "The Journey to Family Well-Being" — a ride where we celebrate triumphs, gain from diversions, and partake simultaneously. It's a section loaded up with accounts of satisfaction, versatility, and the basic delights of being a sound, cheerful family. Welcome to a journey that isn't simply a destination; it's the actual heartbeat of your family's story in 2024 and beyond.

Chapter One:Foundation for Health

So we're starting this trip in "Family Health 2024" with talking about the fundamentals—the things that constitute the firm foundation for your family's well-being. Consider it like constructing a house. You wouldn't construct on shaky ground, would you? This chapter is all about laying the groundwork for a healthier lifestyle that fits your family like a glove. We're not talking about drastic changes here; rather, it's about incorporating good behaviors into your daily routine.

First and foremost, we'll look at habits. Not the intimidating, all-or-nothing sort, but the kind that makes wellness a natural part of your daily routine. Consider this to be the creation of a lifestyle in which being healthy is not a chore but simply the way you roll.

Then we're going to the kitchen. We're not talking about gourmet meals here, but rather basic, conscious choices that ensure your family's bodies and minds receive what they require. It's like filling up your car with nice things to keep it running properly.

But we're not just interested in what's on the menu; we're also curious about how feeling good physically relates to feeling good emotionally. They're like best friends, and we're making sure they're both in great form.

There are no hard and fast rules here. This is about determining what resonates with your family—what connects with your beliefs and dreams. We're not looking for perfection; we're looking for progress, and we know that modest steps add up to great improvements.

So brace yourself for some practical advice, engaging anecdotes, and recommendations that simply make sense. This chapter isn't about changing your health; it's about laying the groundwork for a vibrant family life in 2024 and beyond. Welcome to a chapter where health is about more than just checking boxes.

Establishing Healthy Habits

Okay, buckle up because we're about to get into the phase where healthy living becomes second nature—Establishing Healthy Habits. Consider it establishing a comfortable habit rather than turning your world upside down. Consider this: morning stretches that become your family's daily groove, or swapping out sugary foods in the afternoon for something a little more healthful. These are the subtle changes that, like a favorite music playing in the background, make health a normal part of your day.

We understand; life is already a juggling act, and we're not going to add to it. Instead, we're looking for behaviors that will fit seamlessly into your everyday routine. It's not about turning your life into a health boot camp; it's about developing habits that seem like they've always been there.

As we examine the art of creating habits that stick, expect some practical ideas, real-life anecdotes that you might nod along to, and a few "aha" moments. This is not a race; it is a slow and steady trek towards a better, happier family life. So prepare for a journey in which choosing healthy choices will no longer feel like a chore. "Establishing Healthy Habits" is where health becomes a groove, a vibe, and a natural part of your family's journey in 2024 and beyond. Let's make this habit thing a piece of cake!

A healthy, active lifestyle can aid in weight maintenance and the prevention of health problems such as diabetes, heart disease, asthma, and high blood pressure. If you have a family, it is critical to keep them healthy and happy as well. However, raising a family is not always simple. You and your children are both quite busy.

Early on, there are several simple strategies to instill healthy behaviors and wise decisions in your family.

Here are 12 suggestions to help you and your family live a healthy and happy life:

1. Workout.

Have a friendly competition to see who can do the most pushups, hold a plank the longest, or do the most jumping jacks during commercial breaks or between Netflix episodes. Play is beneficial to the health of your family.

2. Be willing to forgive.

Make mistakes in front of your children and seek forgiveness. By modeling this behavior, you may improve your personal health and well-being while also teaching your children to let go of grudges and resentment.

3. Control your servings.

Every meal should include fruits and vegetables. Make fruits and vegetables available to children without forcing them to consume them. Make healthy eating a priority. Your children are watching.

4. Take an active role in your health treatment.

Maintain a schedule for well-child visits. These appointments are used to monitor your child's growth, behaviour, sleep, eating habits, and social development.

5. Get enough rest.

Sleep is a vital component of children's success. Aim for an early bedtime and a consistent evening routine that includes no screen time. Remember that sleep-deprived youngsters frequently wind up rather than slow down.

6. Experiment with new things.

Make a list of activities you'd like to try as a family and post it somewhere everyone can see it.

7. Increase your strength.

Strength and flexibility should be included in your family's physical activity regimen. Stretching during commercials or doing calf raises while brushing teeth are two examples.

8. Look for joy.

Every day, find something to chuckle about with your family. Laughter relieves stress and anxiety.

9. Spend time with family and friends.

By being kind to your loved ones, you may instill the value of developing solid relationships. Children will learn that giving, rather than receiving, can bring true satisfaction. Schedule regular virtual time with loved ones who live elsewhere.

10. Get rid of your addictions.

Make screen time a privilege that can be used only after chores and homework have been accomplished. Limit your child's screen usage to no more than two hours each day, and keep screens out of his or her bedroom.

11. Reduce your stress.

Look for free yoga videos for kids and families online, or try incorporating deep breathing into your kids' sleep routine. Children, like adults, endure stress and anxiety.

12. Express thankfulness.

Make a gratitude jar and urge everyone to place a note in it every day with something they are thankful for. Take some time to read them while everyone is at the dinner table. During difficult moments, open your heart to thankfulness and acknowledge your sorrow.

If you're having trouble convincing your family to adopt healthy habits, remember that modeling healthy behaviors is an excellent place to start. You may not be able to influence your family's behavior, but you may begin your own wellness path. When they see the changes you're making, odds are they'll want to join you.

Nourishing Your Family's Body and Mind

Hello there! So let's get started in "Family Health 2024" with a discussion about "Nourishing Your Family's Body and Mind." Consider this part to be your favorite cozy kitchen, where the heart of your family's well-being is prepared. Okay, we're not going to go on a crazy diet or urge you to give up all your comfort foods. No, we're talking about the good stuff—food that not only keeps your bodies going but also adds a little joy to your family moments.

Consider substituting colorful fruits for manufactured snacks, or turning dinner into a time to share tales and laugh. These aren't simply meals; they're moments that fill more than your stomachs; they strengthen your family relationships.

Life may be unpredictable, right? It's okay if not every night is a gourmet dinner night. We're figuring out how to include healthy eating into your daily routine, whether you're a skilled cook or a takeaway junkie.

Get ready for some down-to-earth advice, stories that will make you laugh, and maybe even a dish that will become your family's new favorite. This isn't about food regulations; it's about establishing an atmosphere in which feeding your family becomes a pleasure rather than a work. So come on in and take a seat at the virtual kitchen table. Welcome to the discussion on "Nourishing Your Family's Body and Mind." It's a journey in which each mouthful leads to a better, happier family life. Let's make feeding your family a delicious adventure!

As parents, we try to protect our children from anything that we believe may be damaging to them. We instill in them the importance of safety on the playground and during other outside activities; we tell them about the dangers of strangers;

and we use caution when crossing the street. However, how much do we truly care about what kids eat and how well they are nourished? Of course, we want our children to have three meals a day, enough food and drink, and not go hungry, but do we really care if they have eight glasses of water, five servings of fruits and vegetables, five servings of grains, and so on? Most of the time, the answer is "No." We adore our children, without a doubt, but we just do not devote enough time or attention to ensuring that they receive the correct amount of each meal type that they require.

Whether you're a kid or a teen: Having a Good Time with Nutrition

It is our obligation, regardless of age, to ensure our children's health and well-being while they are under our care and supervision. One way to do this is to ensure that kids are eating healthily and understand the importance of appropriate nutrition. When our children are toddlers, this appears to provide a completely different set of challenges. Young children are picky about food's flavors, textures, and colors. They dislike trying new things. According to some studies, a child may require up to eighteen suggestions or attempts before they will try anything new. As a parent, this can be time-consuming and annoying.

We can try the following strategies to encourage our toddlers to absorb their colors, shapes, textures, and everything in between:

1. Eat meals together: When a family eats together, they are more likely to enjoy a variety of foods, and if everyone else is eating something, the kids are more likely to eat it as well, particularly broccoli or whole-wheat buns. Not to add that when you're talking, everything tastes better.

2. As a parent and a cook, conceal as many foods as possible. Serve whole wheat pasta instead of semolina, and purée spinach in your spaghetti sauce whenever possible. If you are as creative as you can and should be, your family will obtain the required vitamins and minerals, and you will have fewer disputes with the kids.

3. Provide diversity as soon as possible, whenever possible. As a child grows older, he may become more set in his ways. Children are incredible creatures of habit. For example, if a child discovers he or she is infatuated with mac and cheese, they may decide that's all they want to eat for the next two months. They are more likely to avoid adhering to a single cuisine if you introduce them to a variety of meals and they are eager "to bite." As a result, they will be able to significantly increase their nutrition.

4. Set a good example. When our children see us eating fruits and vegetables, drinking eight glasses of water, and choosing frozen yogurt over ice cream, they will understand the importance of taking care of their health. More importantly, we can teach kids the importance of taking care of their bodies. Better yet, we may impart the value of moderation in children at a young age by educating them to avoid squandering anything and overindulging.

Food Play for Toddlers

Involving older children and teenagers in meal preparation increases their interest in nutrition and eating. When children are between the ages of five and ten, parents can encourage them to help with simple tasks such as these:

1. Meal planning. Find out what your child wants to eat for dinner with the family or for lunch at school. Give them two or three choices and ask them to pick one. They should choose a grain, a protein, and a fruit or vegetable. Inform them about the significance and necessity of the numerous food types that our bodies require.

2. Involve your children in the preparation process whenever possible, and make it enjoyable for them. They may wash the rice and cut the vegetables themselves, and they can even measure and pour the seasonings directly into the saucepan. If you keep an eye on them, they can use the mixer or blender to blend or puree food.

3. Add some levity to your cuisine. If you're having pizza for dinner, make little pizzas. Purchase miniature dough and allow the kids to make their own pizzas. Arrange the cheese, sauce, and toppings, and then let your creativity run wild. When a child makes her own pizza, you'll be astonished at how many vegetables she consumes—of course, they must assist with cleanup.

Teaching Teens Nutritional Fundamentals

Teens are capable of much more than just grating cheese and slicing onions for you. Instead than telling them what's for dinner, why don't you let them choose?

Allow them to cook dinner from scratch one or two nights a week when they don't have as much coursework to finish. This can include deciding what to make, giving you a shopping list of the ingredients they'll need (or shopping alone), preparing the supper (with or without your help), and serving it. Indeed, we must grant them permission to use our exquisite delicacies!

Teens will have formed the majority of their manners and behaviors related to raising their own children by this age.

Allow them to 'practice' in your home before they buy one so they understand the importance of well-balanced meals, healthy eating, family meals and gracious hospitality. We should train them not only to prepare healthy meals for their families and themselves, but also to do so swiftly, inexpensively, gracefully, and with the best of intentions. This suggests that individuals must evaluate their way of life, enjoyment, health, and etiquette.

We must infuse etiquette and politeness into every part of our lives. To remember people who do not have as much as we do, we must remember to give thanks before meals, express thankfulness after each meal, regularly donate to organizations, and avoid wasting or throwing food. There are specific etiquette and manners that we should observe when eating and drinking.

We teach these manners to our children, and it is our obligation to teach them how to observe them, remember them when the time comes, and then teach their own families when the time comes. As parents, we have a responsibility to show our children the importance of taking care of and respecting our bodies, in addition to eating nutritious food. We educate our children to respect our bodies and minds by exercising, eating healthily, worshiping, and expressing thanks when appropriate. This will benefit our children even beyond their formative years, providing them with a lifetime of happy and nutritious experiences.

CHAPTER Two:Fitness Fusion

So we're dancing to the beat of "Fitness Fusion" in "Family Health 2024."

Consider this chapter to be a joyful mixtape in which fitness becomes a family

affair without the dull gym atmosphere. Let's forget about hard-core workouts

and instead focus on making movement a celebration. Consider it a dance floor

where each family member can choose their favorite moves. It's about finding

delight in being active together, turning fitness into a chance to have fun and feel

good. We're looking into exercises that don't feel like punishment. Consider

stretching in the morning that feels more like a group embrace or turning your

living room into a dance party. These are the types of workouts that leave you

feeling energized rather than exhausted.

Isn't life hectic right now? So we're working out how to get some movement in

without stressing ourselves out. It's all about turning mundane activities into

chances to get those bodies moving. There's no pressure, just a little fun. Expect

some practical advice, maybe a funny anecdote or two, and stories about families finding their fitness groove. It's not about being gym rats; it's about developing a fitness attitude that fits your family's personality.

So, whether it's backyard yoga, a stroll around the park, or a full-on family dance-off in the living room, welcome to "Fitness Fusion." It's a chapter where working out is motivated by joy rather than responsibility, as you celebrate your family's vitality in 2024 and beyond. Prepare to move, groove, and enjoy the workout fun!

Fun and Effective Workouts for All Ages

Let's talk about making exercise something the whole family can enjoy in "Family Health 2024." This part of chapter two is devoted to "Fun and Effective Workouts for People of All Ages." And believe me, it's not about dragging everyone to a punishing workout—it's about making exercise fun. Consider this a workout celebration for the entire family, from toddlers to seasoned athletes. We're talking about workouts that don't seem like a chore, but rather like fun. Consider making your living room into a tiny adventure area, or turning a stroll around the park into a scavenger hunt. These workouts are designed to make you smile rather than groan.

Here's the cool part: we understand that everyone is unique. So, whether your family enjoys dance-offs, family yoga sessions, or making household duties a workout, we've got you covered.

Isn't it true that life may be a whirlwind? As a result, we're keeping everything real and realistic. These routines fit perfectly into your family's schedule, making fitness feel less like a chore and more like a shared experience.

Prepare for some amusing advice, a few laughs, and anecdotes about families finding their groove together. We're not going for a sweaty mess here; we're going for a nice time, a bonding experience that brings your family closer together. Welcome to a chapter where working out isn't a requirement; rather, it's a celebration of your family's zest for life in 2024 and beyond. Prepare to move and have fun on the journey!

Exercise Advantages for Your Family

Enhances Memory

- Anaerobic exercise increases verbal memory and thinking, according to a study conducted at the University of British Columbia.

Reduces Anxiety and Improves Mood

- Many people experience a mood increase five minutes after moderate activity. According to research, these feelings can have long-term consequences. According to one study, exercise and antidepressants are both effective treatments for severe depressive illness.

- Another study discovered that exercise can lessen anxiety sensitivity and aid in preventing panic episodes.

Lowers the risk of cardiovascular disease and other chronic diseases

- Physical activity has been demonstrated in studies to reduce the risk of cardiovascular disease and several other chronic illnesses, such as diabetes, cancer, hypertension, obesity, and osteoporosis.

The Value of Family Fitness

Maintain Your Health Together

- Create healthy habits in your child by getting them active at an early age. Working out jointly allows you to reap the above-mentioned health benefits.

Take advantage of Family Bonding Time

- It might be difficult to integrate family time and physical activity into your family's busy schedule between school, work, and playdates. Active play contributes to the strengthening of family relationships, which is essential for your child's social and emotional development. Plus, you all get the daily activity you need at the same time!.

20 Family-Friendly Active Workout Activities

1. Make it into a game. Using regular playing cards, make a deck of fitness training cards. Hearts represent push-ups, clubs represent crunches, diamonds represent jumping jacks, and spades represent squats. Allow your youngster to choose a card and then complete as many of the activities listed on the card. For instance, an ace of spades equals one squat and a six of hearts equals six pushups.

2. Play Take turns following the Leader through a variety of activities (skipping, jumping, marching, etc.). Alternatively, take turns acting as the "coach" and telling the "athlete" what to do.

3. Take a walk. You can incorporate walks into your everyday routine before or after dinner. Allow smaller children to alternate between riding in a pram or waggon and walking. Bring your dogs to make it more enjoyable. Alternatively, go on a walk with your older children.

4. Ride your bike to the library, the grocery store, or the park. Once at the park, you can have a picnic or engage in an energetic activity such as frisbee or kite flying. To prevent dragging a bike and a child back home, keep track of the distance you're riding and turn around before your child becomes tired. Use scooters or roller skates instead of bikes if your child wants to try something new.

5. Take some active play to the playground. Your neighborhood playground has monkey bars, rock climbing walls, swings, and more. Whether you play "Lava" or just run about, the park is a great place to get some exercise.

6. Is it raining? Let's go bowling! Even small children can bowl with the help of bumpers and a bowling ramp. Or they can practice at home with a foam or plastic bowling set.

7. Play sports in your backyard with your family or other neighborhood youngsters. Basketball, soccer, baseball, and flag

football are all entertaining options. If you don't have enough participants, you can modify the game, concentrate on sport-specific abilities (like throwing or dribbling), or find more in a community center. If your child enjoys a sport, consider coaching the team to mix family time and exercise.

8. Make time to enjoy traditional outdoor activities. Hide and seek, kick the can, kickball, hopscotch, tag, jump rope, and other childhood activities can all be introduced to your children as active games.

9. Let's have a dance party! Turn on the music and start dancing about the living room. For added ambiance, use a disco ball or freeze dance. If your family enjoys dancing, consider enrolling in a formal dance class. Family dance classes are available at some studios. Alternatively, you might take an adult class at the same time as your child's session and teach each other the moves at home.

10. Stick with a tried-and-true alternative and head outside to play catch. If your youngster needs more practice, have them stand close together and take a step back after each successful catch.

11. If no one in your family has a favorite exercise activity, try something new once a week. It's a terrific opportunity to switch things up and discover something you all enjoy, whether it's ice skating, rock climbing or going on a walk.

12. Try a workout class if you work better with a set schedule. It incorporates fitness into your family's weekly routine and provides newcomers with simple directions to follow. Looking for inspiration to get started? Zumba, yoga, kickboxing, and martial arts are all good options.

13. Create your own home gym if you aren't ready to take your children to the gym and keep them from climbing on fitness equipment. Instead, introduce them to kid-friendly exercise equipment such as light free weights, latex-free resistance

bands (the CLX includes loops that are excellent for young hands to handle), and exercise balls, as well as easy activities.

14. Go swimming! Swimming is a terrific low-impact training option whether you're at the beach or at the YMCA. Splash about in the water, teach your child to swim, play Marco Polo, or swim laps.

15. Extend your swimming experience with enjoyable aquatic activities. You'll have a good time whether you're canoeing, kayaking, paddleboarding, surfing, water skiing, wakeboarding, or tubing.

16. Stay active by playing some outdoor games. Croquet, bocce ball, horseshoes, and ring toss are all simple activities that may be enjoyed by people of all ages.

17. Play some mini-golf. Mini golf is a great way to start teaching your child basic golf basics in a fun environment. When your youngster is ready, take him or her to the driving range or a real-world golf course.

18. Make housework an active game. Save the world by sweeping dust bunnies away with a broom or vacuuming them away. Encourage your kids to save their stuffed animals from "floor lava" by racing them to put them away and clean up their room.

19. Run a 5k as a family to stay fit. Most 7-10 year olds can walk/run a 5k at 3.1 miles. To encourage your child interested in running, Disney offers entertaining versions such as color runs, glow runs, and 5ks.

20. Request assistance with yard work from your children. Raking leaves, planting and managing a garden and shoveling snow all raise your heart rate while completing tasks on your family's to-do list.

Family Fitness by Age

Choosing age-appropriate activities is a big component of creating a pleasant and sustainable family fitness programme. Depending on the age of your child(ren), here are some suggestions for your family to consider.

3 to 5 years old

The Centres for Disease Control and Prevention (CDC) recommends that children between the ages of 3 and 5 be "active throughout the day" to enhance their growth and development. Other countries' exercise standards, such as those from Canada and the United Kingdom, recommend three active hours per day for children in this age range.

This does not have to be continuous moderate or strenuous activity, but could include play and physical activities supervised by an adult. The CDC states that "children do not usually need formal muscle-strengthening programmes," but they should also not be idle for long periods of time, unless they are sleeping.

Family exercise activities for children aged 3 to 5 could include:

Having fun on a jungle gym

Gymnastics practice

Tree climbing

Taking part in a game such as "Follow the Leader" or "Duck, Duck, Goose"

Back-and-forth kicking of a ball

The game of freeze tag

Creating an obstacle course

Taking part in a treasure hunt

Catching a ball

Dancing to music in a group

Investigating the backyard

6 to 10 years old

The CDC advises a minimum of 60 minutes of moderate or intense physical exercise every day for children over the age of six. Again, these activities can be short bursts of movement throughout the day, as children's attention spans often require them to engage in one activity quickly before moving on to the next. The majority of daily sessions should consist of aerobic activity, such as walking or running, and at least three days per week should consist of intense activity. Children of this age should also engage in bone and muscle strengthening exercises, such as climbing or jumping.

If your child is in this age range, here are some family fitness activities to consider:

Biking

Riding an unpowered scooter

Participating in baseball or softball

Tree climbing or rope climbing

Some types of yoga

Combat sports

Flag football or tag football

Rope jumping

Swimming

Rollerblading

Ages 10+

As your child grows older and becomes a tween, then a teen, the physical activity requirements remain the same. They will still require at least 60 minutes of moderate to strenuous activity each day, with their programme including aerobic, muscle-strengthening, and bone-strengthening activities.

Teenagers, particularly teenage boys, have a predisposition to over-exercise. As a result, engaging in fitness as a family can assist tweens and adolescents in learning healthy behaviors as well as how to exercise safely and effectively.

Here are some family fitness activities for kids aged 10 and above to consider:

Hiking

Running, possibly in preparation for a charity run

Biking

Kayaking

Housework and garden work, such as grass mowing

Skiing in the cross-country course

Body weight or weighted resistance exercises

Skateboarding

Football and volleyball are examples of team sports.

Making baskets

Throwing a frisbee

Attending dancing classes

Building a Strong and Active Family

A secure and joyful home environment is essential for both physical and mental health. In today's fast-paced world, it is critical to remember that your family is your primary source of support and affection. Celebrating accomplishments or significant milestones with family members adds meaning to your life. A strong family life also provides stability throughout stressful times and life transitions.

Do Activities as a Family

Family activities promote interaction and serve to develop communication among all members of the family. Plan regular family visits to areas like the park, beach, or museum, volunteer together to participate in community events, or plan family vacation itineraries together.

Establishing family rituals and customs also contributes to the creation of a supportive and caring environment. These routines can be done on a regular basis and can be as basic as setting aside time for family dinners or discussing each other's days with the family. You might also involve your children in domestic duties and create a roster for everyone in the family to participate. Celebrating anniversaries, family reunions, or other festivals such as Chinese New Year, Hari Raya, or Deepavali together are all excellent opportunities to include family customs.

Family routines and customs help to form younger family members' sense of commitment and responsibility, as well as further shape a family's identity. Spending time together also helps each person develop a sense of belonging and fosters sentiments of familiarity, understanding, and trust. When you have a strong foundation of relationships, you will be able to identify when someone is not acting normally and provide attention and support more immediately.

Personal Confidence and Trust Within the Family

Aside from group conversation and interaction, it is also critical to reinforce the individual bonds that comprise the family unit. Spending frequent one-on-one time would help to create the connection and trust needed in a healthy family. These sessions could take place between a parent and a child, between a grandmother and a youngster, or between siblings.

Aside from offering to listen and understand, one-on-one sharing allows you to share your experiences and learning with other family members. During such meetings, it is also critical to be patient and supportive. You could encourage nonjudgmental sharing of thoughts, feelings, and issues. You would be able to recognise difficulties earlier and prevent them from growing further if you spoke often.

Be there for one another.

Dad has received a promotion in his career. Daughter received As on all of her exams. Mum has been named Mother of the Year. There are examples of joyful events that should be shared with one another, particularly with family. It's a terrific moment to congratulate and celebrate one another's accomplishments.

When successes are shared with family and loved ones, happiness increases. The highs of life should be recognised, and this is an excellent occasion to express gratitude to your family members who have contributed to your achievement in any way.

Life might also be challenging at times due to obligations at work or school. In these moments, one must be careful not to keep these difficulties to themselves. The additional stress and irritation can have a bad affect on your family and your connection with them.

Learn to take a courageous step forward in times of adversity to seek their assistance and support. A listening ear can ease feelings of loneliness. Be open to the possibility that someone else will come up with brilliant solutions to your problems. Difficult circumstances are simpler to get through with the help of your family rather than facing them alone.

Tips

Participating in family routines and customs can assist to create an environment that promotes mental health. These can be as simple as eating meals together on a regular basis or going on family vacations.

It is critical to spend one-on-one time with each member of the family in order to create trust and share burdens.

Family emotional support can assist relieve stress.

Chapter 3: Mindful Nutrition

Consider this chapter to be a friendly discussion about making food more than just fuel. We're delving into the concept of mindful choices, or paying attention not only to what you consume but also to how it makes you feel.

Imagine sitting down to a meal and truly experiencing each bite, savoring the flavors, colors, and textures. It's not about following rigid rules or counting calories; it's about developing a mindset in which food is a source of joy and sustenance.

Isn't life getting insane now? So mindful nutrition does not need spending hours in the kitchen or obsessing over every meal. It's about finding easy ways to pay attention to what you eat, whether it's a family dinner or a short snack.

Expect some simple advice, relatable tales, and even a recipe or two to make mindful eating a breeze. This isn't about giving up items you enjoy; it's about developing a healthy relationship with food that benefits your entire family.

One of the most frequently asked questions at our mindful eating events is how to teach youngsters about mindful eating and practice it during family meals. Everyone should practice mindfulness when cooking and dining together as a family.

Young children have an internal dietician who advises them on what and how much to eat. Little children who are given a range of foods on their high chair tray will eat the appropriate sorts and amounts of each food. The catch is that they will not eat in a balanced manner in a single day, but rather throughout a week. We can only imagine how soon this natural eating style will be interrupted. Parents notice that their child has only eaten mashed potatoes one day and applesauce the next. Concerned that their child is not getting enough protein, parents start interfering, cajoling, bribing, and attempting to force food into the infant's closed mouth. According to studies, at the age of five, children will heroically attempt to consume the entire serving of macaroni and cheese.

Thus begins our particularly American practice of attempting to wipe our plates at "family style" restaurants where large servings of cheap food are regarded as "a good deal." We are even taught that if we don't eat it all, we are somehow contributing to the plight of starving children in Africa. Mindful eating allows us to reconnect with the advice of our internal dietician.

How can parents teach their children about mindful eating? Here are a few ideas.

- Every day, have at least one pleasant family meal. When the environment is pleasant and everyone discusses their day's activities, youngsters learn to eat deliberately and to associate eating with delight and connection. Eating and anxiety are not a good combination. Eating and feeling at ease are.

- Allow children to assist you in preparing the dinner. Discuss where each piece of food comes from and how the Earth, sun, rain, and many individuals contributed to its arrival at your table.

- Start family dinners with a simple grace. It might be as simple as simply joining hands and bowing heads around the table to recall and thank the many people and creatures who brought the food to the table. Pausing teaches children not to run away from their meal.

- Experiment with different foods and beverages. Fresh apricots, pineapple, or dates are all good options. Purchase persimmon, papaya, mango, kiwi, star fruit, or red bananas from an ethnic grocery store; tamarind, guava, or coconut juice. "This is a fruit that children in (Mexico, Japan, Thailand, etc.) enjoy eating." Take a whiff of it. What is the fragrance like? Take a small bite or sip and tell me how it tastes." Experimentation allows children to discover the enormous world of varied flavors rather than becoming trapped in a diet of boxed macaroni and canned ravioli.

- Use your imagination when it comes to food. When one boy's mother informed him that broccoli is trees that dinosaurs eat, he told his entire elementary school class about it, and every child began to like eating broccoli.

- Discuss the advantages that each food provides. Milk, cheese, and spinach, for example, contain calcium, which helps to create strong teeth and bones.

- Try out the "how full is my stomach" game. Request that youngsters check in with their stomachs before, midway during, and at the end of a meal. Is it empty, half filled, or completely full? This allows them (and you) to keep in touch with your body's signals of fullness and avoid overeating.

- Avoid discussing calorie counts or restricted diets with children. According to research, females who start dieting as preteens have a substantially increased risk of developing eating disorders. Don't be too strict when it comes to junk food. It is not a tragedy if your children have been raised on home-cooked organic cuisine and enjoy a McDonald's cheeseburger and cola at a birthday celebration. It's an international experience.

- Assist youngsters in distinguishing between bodily hunger and emotions such as boredom, exhaustion, and anxiety. Help children learn to deal with these feelings through activities like exercising, playing a game, reading a book, making crafts, and interacting with friends.

- Holidays and significant occasions should be celebrated. Allow children to assist in the planning of a party. Place a tablecloth, a candle, and flowers on the table. They can make basic decorations out of paper, such as hearts, stars, or Easter eggs. When we treat ourselves as guests, we add a crucial element to the food: an extra scoop of affection.

- The greatest desire of everyone is for love and connection. Our health depends on loving words. Loving words are an alternative method of feeding the heart that does not include food. Give your family and friends big helpings of real expressions of thanks and warm words if you want them to feel well fed. "I really appreciate your ..." "When I am with you I feel ..."

Eating as a family, pausing, slowing down, having fun, experimenting, being interested, exploring new tastes, and adding the flavors of compassion and love to your meals are all part of mindful eating in a family.

Supercharge Your Plate with Nutrient-Rich Delights

Few things in the world of nutrition capture the essence of vitality and well-being more than the vibrant colors and enticing flavors of fresh, nutritious fruits and vegetables. These natural treasures are not only a visual and sensory feast, but also a tremendous source of nourishment for the body and soul. As we embark on a journey of wellness on a plate, we explore the incredible benefits and pleasures that come from including an abundance of nutrient-rich fruits and vegetables in our meals.

The Colorful Nutrient Palette

The rainbow of hues present in fruits and vegetables attests to the wide variety of nutrients they contain. Each color represents a distinct combination of vitamins, minerals, antioxidants, and phytochemicals that contribute to our overall health.

- Red and pink: These colors are frequently associated with the presence of lycopene and anthocyanins, which are known for their antioxidant effects. Tomatoes, watermelon, and strawberries are a few examples.

- Orange and Yellow:Carotenoids such as beta-carotene and zeaxanthin give fruits and vegetables their brilliant orange and yellow hues. Carotenoids help to maintain good vision, immunological function, and skin health. Consider the following vegetables: carrots, sweet potatoes, and bell peppers.

- Green: Chlorophyll-rich leafy greens and cruciferous vegetables are high in fiber and a variety of vitamins and minerals. These nutrient powerhouses aid with cleansing, digestion, and overall well-being.

- Blue and purple: These colors are derived from anthocyanins, which are powerful antioxidants associated to heart health, cognitive function, and inflammation reduction. This group includes blueberries, eggplants, and blackberries.

- White: White fruits and vegetables, such as garlic, onions, and cauliflower, contain allicin and other bioactive components that help the immune system and are anti-inflammatory.

Body and Mind Nutrition

When we incorporate a variety of healthful fruits and vegetables into our meals, we go on a wellness journey that extends far beyond physical nourishment. The nutrients in these foods have an important function in supporting many elements of human health:

- Fruits and vegetables high in antioxidants, fiber, and healthy fats promote cardiovascular health by lowering blood pressure, cholesterol levels, and promoting optimal blood vessel function.

- Gut Health: Vegetable fiber promotes a diversified and flourishing gut microbiota, aiding digestion, nutrient absorption, and a strong immune system.

Antioxidants and phytochemicals present in colorful food have been linked to improved cognitive function and a lower risk of neurodegenerative illnesses.

- Energy and Vitality: Nutrient-dense fruits and vegetables contain vitamins and minerals that help with energy production, immunological support, and general vitality.

- Skin Radiance: The vitamins and antioxidants found in fruits and vegetables help to maintain healthy, glowing skin by guarding against oxidative stress and encouraging collagen development.

The phrase "you are what you eat" could not be more accurate in the pursuit of a healthier lifestyle. As we navigate the busy aisles of grocery shops, it's critical that we pick choices that not only satisfy our taste buds but also provide our bodies with the nutrition they require. This is where the concept of superfoods comes into play: nutrient-dense foods that provide health advantages in addition to basic nutritional value. We go into the world of these nutritious powerhouses that can energize your plate and boost your general well-being in this examination of nutrient-rich superfoods.

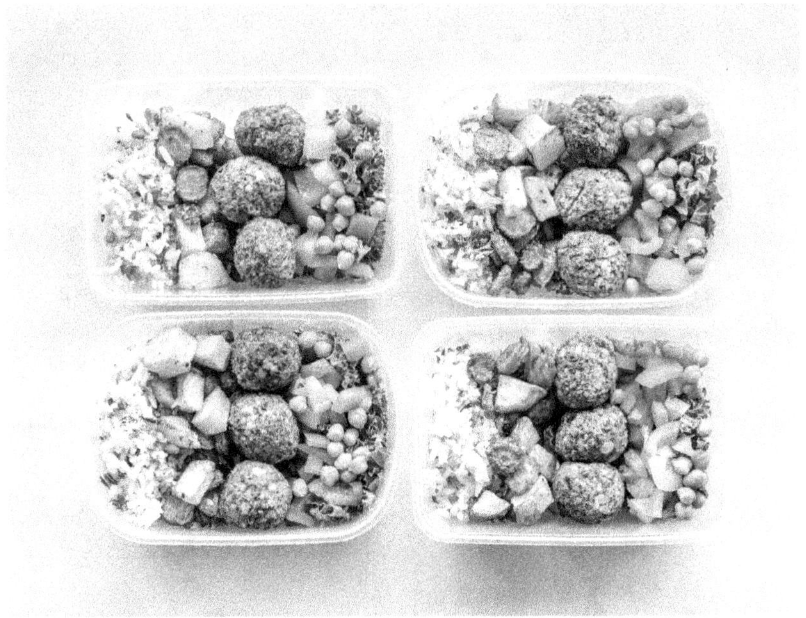

1. Blueberries Are Little Giants

Let's start simple: blueberries. Don't be misled by their little size; these berries are high in antioxidants, vitamins, and fiber. Blueberries have been shown to boost memory and lessen the risk of chronic diseases such as heart disease and diabetes. Add a handful of these colorful berries to your morning oatmeal or yogurt for a tasty and nutritious start to your day.

2. Quinoa: The Whole Protein

Move over, rice; quinoa has arrived to take your place. This ancient grain is not only high in protein, but it also includes all nine necessary amino acids, making it an excellent vegetarian and vegan protein source. Quinoa is also high in fiber, iron, magnesium, and B vitamins. Quinoa is a versatile superfood that can easily become a mainstay in your diet, whether used in salads, bowls, or as a side dish.

3. The King of Greens, Kale

Kale has a well-deserved reputation as a nutritional powerhouse. Kale, which is high in vitamins A, C, and K as well as calcium, provides a variety of health benefits such as strong bones, enhanced vision, and immune system support.

What's the best part? It comes in a variety of forms, from salads and smoothies to crispy kale chips.

4. Salmon is an Omega-3-rich delicacy.

When it comes to sea superfoods, salmon reigns top. This fatty fish is high in omega-3 fatty acids, which are thought to protect the heart. Omega-3 fatty acids also promote brain health and prevent inflammation. Incorporating salmon into your diet a couple of times per week can improve your general health.

5. Chia Seeds: Small Seeds, Huge Benefits

Chia seeds are little, but their nutritional advantages are not. These seeds are high in fiber, omega-3 fatty acids, and plant-based protein. They also have the unusual ability to absorb liquid and develop a gel-like consistency, which makes them an excellent addition to puddings, smoothies, and even as an egg substitute in baking.

6. Sweet potatoes are naturally sweet and high in nutrients.

Replace normal potatoes with their nutrient-dense cousin, sweet potatoes. Sweet potatoes, which are high in beta-carotene, vitamin C, and fiber, not only taste good but also help with skin health, immunity, and digestion. For a filling and nutritious supper, roast, mash, or make fries with them.

7. Greek Yogurt: A Probiotic Superfood

Greek yogurt elevates conventional yogurt by containing more protein and fewer carbs. It's also high in probiotics, which support gut health and aid digestion. It's great as a snack, in smoothies, or as a creamy topping for your morning bowl.

Incorporating these nutrient-dense superfoods into your diet will boost your general health and well-being significantly. However, keep in mind that no single item can give all of the nutrients your body requires. A diversified diet rich in fruits, vegetables, whole grains, lean proteins, and healthy fats is the key to realizing the full potential of these superfoods. So, the next time you go shopping, stock up on these nutritional powerhouses and supercharge your plate for a healthy you!

Snack Smart: Boosting Energy, Suppressing Cravings

We've all experienced that mid-afternoon slump when we feel like we could devour a whole pantry's worth of food. Our bodies are sometimes hungry, and we should consume a proper meal. Other times, however, we simply require an effective snack that will keep us full and our appetite at bay. That is why it is critical to choose your snacks wisely in order to stay on track with your healthy diet.

In fact, there are several foods known as "appetite suppressants" that are excellent for keeping you full and preventing binging on unhealthy snacks. Appetite suppressants are chemicals that inhibit your hunger sensations, such as foods or supplements.

Here is a list of some of the top appetite suppressants that you can use on a daily basis! Some of them may be things you already enjoy, so it may be as simple as bringing a light snack to satisfy those pesky mid-day cravings.

THE SEEDS OF CHIA

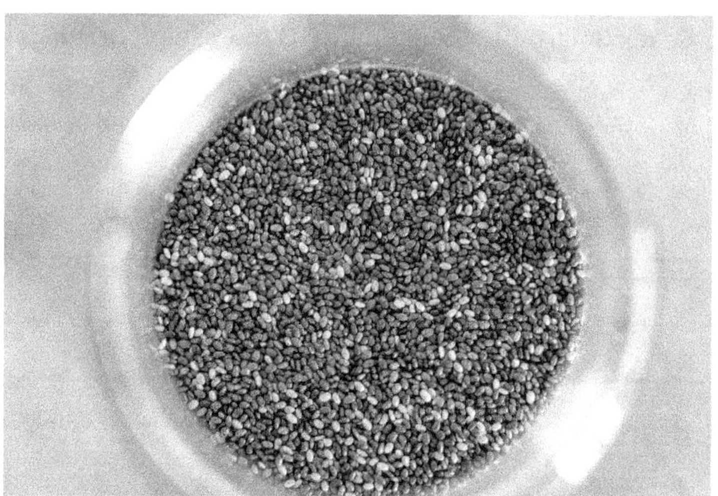

Chia seeds, no matter how little they appear, are nutrient-dense and have appetite-suppressing characteristics. These small snacks are the richest source of plant-based Omega-3 fatty acids. They also have an astonishing amount of soluble fiber. Fiber slows digestion, keeping you fuller for longer.

Chia seeds can also absorb up to ten times their weight in water. As a result, chia seeds absorb a large amount of water, effectively filling you up. Furthermore, they inhibit calorie absorption in the body, lengthening the entire digestive process. Even in modest amounts, chia seeds are extremely effective natural hunger suppressants.

NUTS

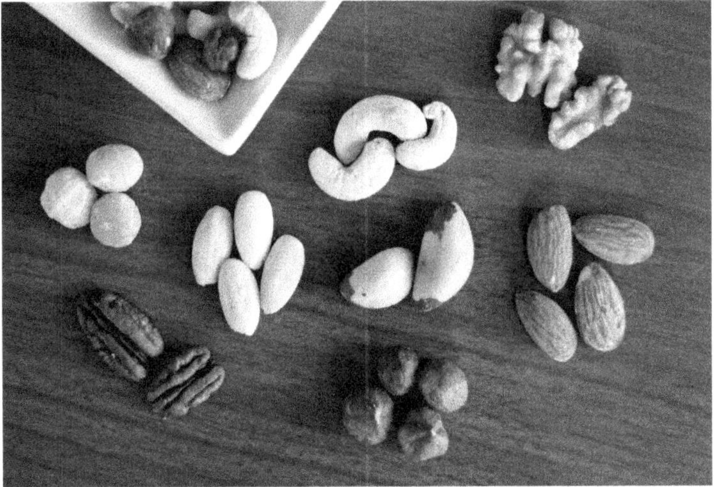

Eating nuts can help you regulate your appetite since the natural healthy fat in them keeps you satisfied for long periods of time. If you are hungry, you can snack on a few nuts or incorporate nuts into your meals so you don't have to eat in between meals. Smoothies can also be made more full by adding a few nuts.

According to a study published in the European Journal of Clinical Nutrition, those who ate 1.5 ounces of almonds per day felt less hungry. Furthermore, because nuts contain a lot of calories, individuals were more conscious and ate less at other times of the day. Walnuts and pine nuts are also high in omega-3 fatty acids, which can help with satiety.

VINEGAR OF APPLE CIDER

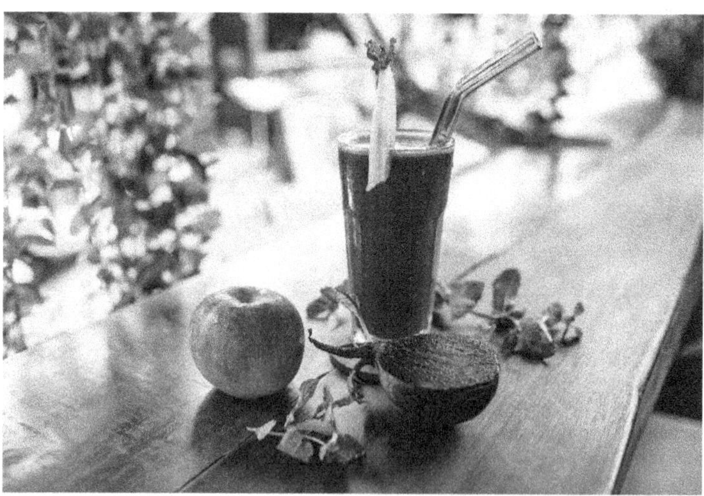

Vinegar, notably Apple Cider Vinegar, has long been used to aid with weight loss.

ACV slows digestion, which keeps you fuller for longer.

ACV is prepared by crushing apples and combining them with yeast, which causes the sugars to ferment into alcohol, which is subsequently fermented into vinegar. ACV also inhibits the body's blood sugar response to meals, resulting in a reduced desire to consume. ACV has been demonstrated in studies to decrease brain areas involved for raising hunger. Other research has found that participants who took apple cider vinegar with a meal felt twice as full as those who did not. AVC is simple to include into salad dressings or dilute in a glass of water. Some folks even begin their day with a shot of it. But be warned: that is not for the faint of heart, and you should be sure you can stomach that much ACV before you try it.

AVOCADO

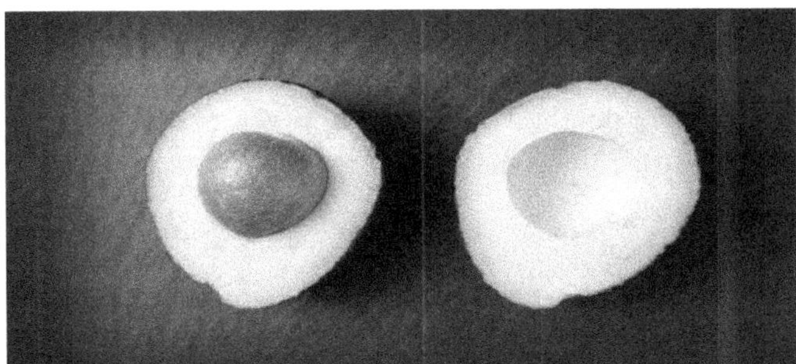

Avocado is abundant in monounsaturated fat and fiber, making it one of the most effective natural hunger suppressants. According to University of California studies, unsaturated fats like oleic acid present in avocados cause your small intestine to manufacture a chemical called oleoylethanolamide. This molecule regulates appetite by connecting with nerve endings; it activates a brain circuit that promotes sensations of fullness, which can aid in the maintenance of a healthy body weight.

CINNAMON

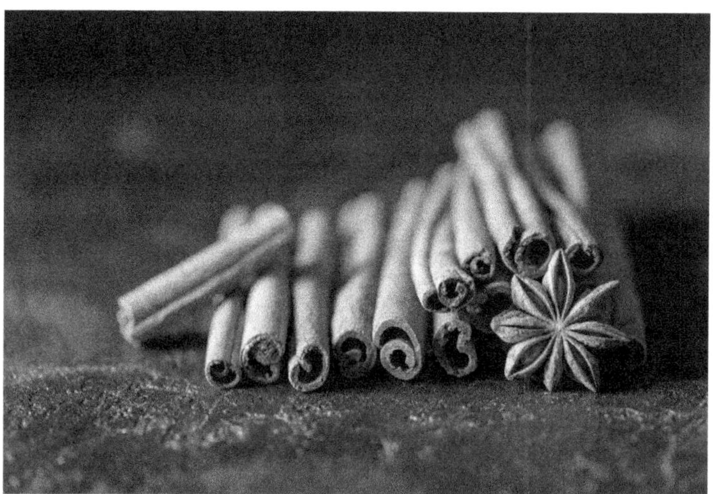

Cinnamon, one of the most potent spices available, acts as an appetite suppressant by regulating blood sugar levels and delaying gastric emptying (the process by which nutrients from your stomach travel into your upper intestine to be absorbed). According to experts published in The American Journal of Clinical Nutrition, cinnamon can really deceive your brain into thinking you are full when you haven't even eaten anything.

Cinnamon is simple to incorporate into meals and drinks. One of our favorite ways to use it is to sprinkle it on a dish of sliced apples. Without the guilt of apple pie! You can use it on a daily basis to keep your hunger under control.

THE GREEN TEA

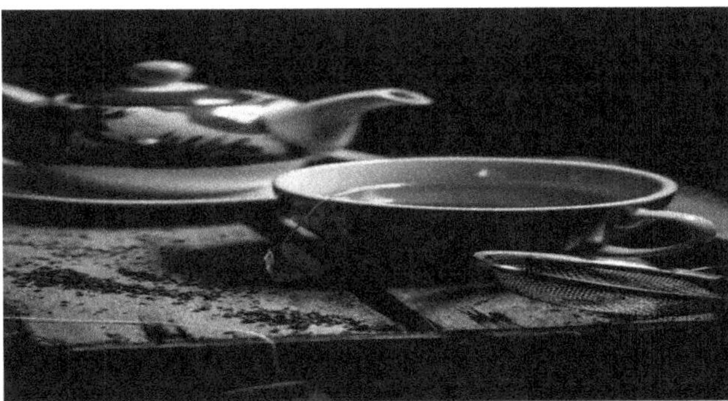

Want to avoid the lunchtime munchies? Make a cup of green tea or mix a couple of spoonfuls of matcha (ground up green tea leaves) into hot water; the caffeine will help you feel full. Green tea also contains fat-burning capabilities, so it will give you a small metabolic boost.

According to a study published in The Journal of Nutrition, people who drank four to five cups of green tea per day and worked out for at least 180 minutes per week lost more stomach fat and total body weight after three months than those who exercised alone.

OATS

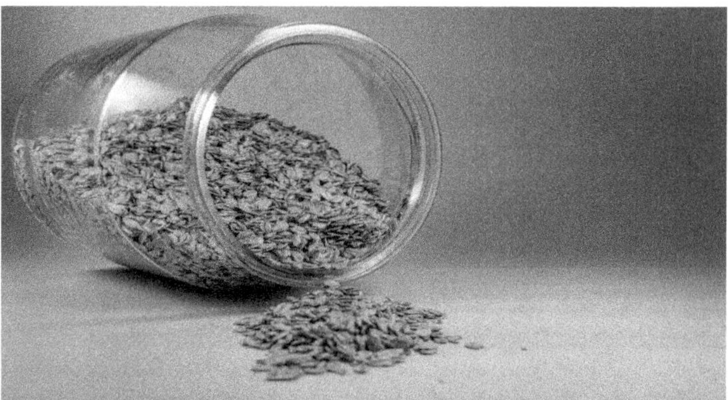

Starting your day with a bowl of thick, healthy oatmeal is one approach to keep yourself satiated until your lunch break. Because oats are a whole grain, they are high in fiber, which allows for a slow breakdown in the gut. This also keeps the feeling of fullness consistent. Dressing oatmeal with extra components like milk and almonds simply increases its protein and fat content, making the meal even more nutritious.

PEPPERMINT

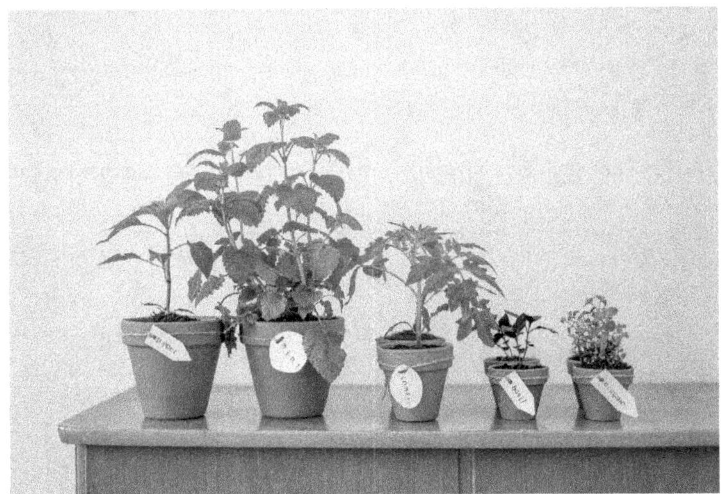

That's true, peppermint is a surprisingly useful solution for hunger reduction and control. Peppermint has long been used in essential oils to relieve tension, but the fragrance can also aid with appetite suppression.

Drinking peppermint tea not only helps curb cravings, but it also boosts your metabolism and improves meal digestion. According to research from Wheeling Jesuit University, those who smelt peppermint every two hours for five days ate 2,800 fewer calories in a week. Isn't this a somewhat odd study? Nonetheless, the data support the hypothesis that including peppermint into your diet could be a good strategy to help you lose weight.

Another study from the University of Rhode Island discovered that chewing gum can lower calorie consumption while increasing energy expenditure.

WATER

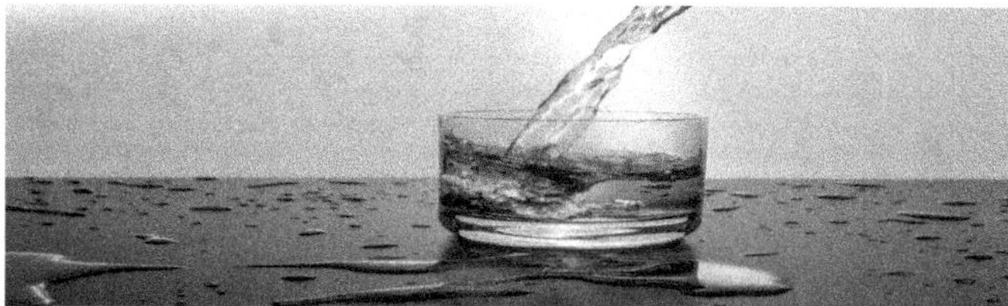

Water is the most simple and easily accessible natural appetite suppressor. That's correct, sometimes all it takes is a glass of cool water. When the body becomes dehydrated, it is common to confuse thirst for hunger. Constant water consumption is required to avoid false hunger feelings.

Furthermore, drinking helps keep the stomach full between meals. This will help you prevent mindless munching and decrease needless desires. Take your water as cold as possible for further benefits; this helps to boost the body's metabolism, resulting in more calories expended.

FOODS WITH SPICES

From chiles to hot sauce and a dash of spicy flavor. Any of these foods will not only satisfy your hunger, but will also boost your body's ability to burn fat (thank you, capsaicin). According to one study, hot chili peppers trigger a nerve in the stomach that tells your body when it's full.

Super-spicy dishes and sauces are also known to slow down how quickly you eat your food. Because your mouth is so heated, you can't consume as quickly, allowing your brain to detect you've eaten enough to eat and preventing overindulgence.

Piperine, also known as black pepper, is another excellent spicy natural appetite suppressant and fat burner. That stuff that comes out of the mill. It has been shown to promote digestion, allowing your metabolism to break down fat more efficiently.

DARK CHOCOLATE

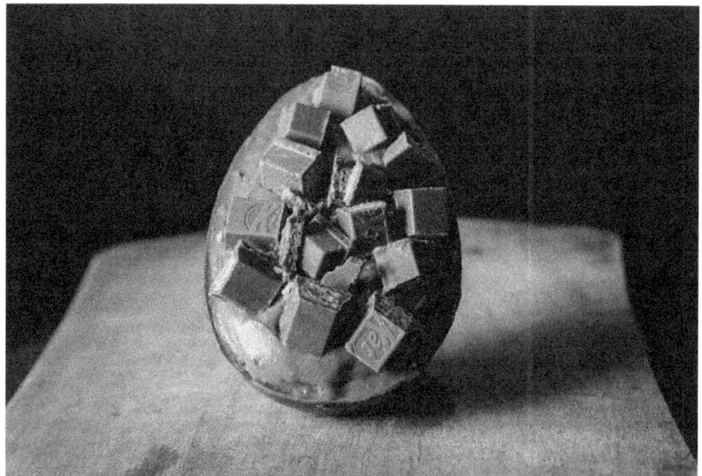

Everyone has a sweet tooth, and quitting sugar is one of the most difficult things to accomplish. However, you do not have to fully eliminate sweets from your life. In fact, eating 70% or higher dark chocolate is excellent for your health. Dark chocolate has a lot of healthy fat and flavonoids, which are phytonutrients. One study published in Nutrition & Diabetes discovered that 100g of dark chocolate increased satiety in men. It also reduced their desire to consume junk food. So it's a win-win situation for everyone.

COFFEE

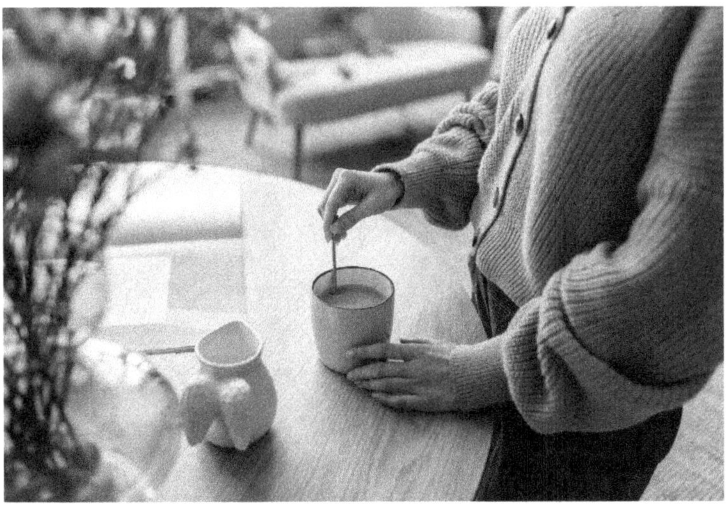

Many individuals cannot fathom their lives without coffee. Fortunately for the numerous coffee addicts out there, this beverage aids with weight control by keeping you fuller for longer. According to studies, caffeine in coffee not only increases your metabolism, but it also keeps your stomach full, minimizing the need to snack.

This does not, however, imply that you should drink coffee all day. Excessive caffeine use, which coffee contains in big quantities, can be hazardous, resulting in adverse effects such as anxiety, hypertension, and agitation.

Chapter 4: Sleep Harmony

This chapter is all about "Sleep Harmony," and believe me when I say it isn't about making sleep a war.

Consider this chapter to be your guide to developing the most cozy, dreamy sleep routine for your family. We're not talking about rigid schedules or sophisticated sleep tactics; we're talking about making bedtime a relaxing routine that everyone enjoys.

Consider your bedroom a sanctuary of tranquility, complete with soft blankets, mild lighting, and perhaps a scent of lavender in the air. It's about making your sleeping area a hideaway, a location where relaxation takes center stage and your body knows it's time to unwind.

Isn't it true that life may be a whirlwind? So, discovering what works for your family is more important than obtaining sleep harmony. It's all about making bedtime a time for connection and rest, from bedtime stories to creating a tech-free zone before sleep.

Expect some practical advice, perhaps a recipe for a cozy sleep-inducing drink, and anecdotes about families discovering the enchantment of a good night's sleep.

This isn't about foregoing midnight pleasure; it's about ensuring that everyone, from the kids to the adults, gets enough rest for the next day's adventures.

So, here's to "Sleep Harmony"—a chapter in 2024 and beyond where sleep isn't a battleground but a peaceful trip for your family. Prepare to be enchanted by the enchantment of beautiful dreams and awaken to brighter mornings!

The Sleep Science

You may not remember everything that occurs as you fall asleep each night, but a lot is happening in your brain and body. Every body system experiences alterations between sleep and wake periods, but none are as significant as changes in consciousness when sleeping.

"Like wakefulness, sleep (both NREM and REM) is a dynamic process regulated by a complex, and only partially understood, network of neural pathways from the brainstem to the cerebral cortex. "Like waking functions, sleep is a developmental process that changes throughout our lives, from infancy to old age."

The Different Sleep Stages

The brain cycles through numerous phases of sleep on a regular basis, and the brain's activity alters as it moves between various sleep stages.

First stage of non-REM (rapid eye movement).

The first stage is when you fall asleep - this is known as non-REM stage 1. Your heart rate, breathing rate, and eye movement all calm down, and your muscles begin to relax. Your brain waves slow down as well, therefore getting up at this early stage of sleep is still pretty easy.

Second stage of non-REM sleep

Your heart rate and body temperature both decrease in the second stage. Except for brief bursts of activity, eye movement ceases completely and your brain slows drastically, while brief bursts of activity let you sleep regardless of outside disturbances.

Third stage of non-REM sleep

Deep slumber ensues. This is an important and critical step. Your heart rate and respiration rate are the lowest during this stage of sleep, making it difficult to wake up. Delta waves characterize brain activity at this period.

REM sleep

Though dreams can occur at any stage of sleep, they are more common during the dream state. Finally, REM sleep occurs when your eyes dart back and forth from side to side (while your eyelids remain closed). Brain activity rises substantially, reaching that of being awake.

Your breathing becomes quicker and more irregular during REM sleep. Although your heart rate and blood pressure continue to return to normal, your arm and leg muscles become temporarily immobile. According to sleep scientists, this paralysis is a protection mechanism that our bodies evolved to protect us from damage or other harm that could come if we "acted out" our dreams. currently arrow

Each sleep cycle (the sum of all stages) lasts around 90 minutes. During each cycle, most people spend more time in deeper sleep earlier in the night — and more time in REM sleep later in the night. Sleep is crucial for numerous learning and memory consolidation processes, and each stage of sleep is vital and profound.

Unlocking the Secrets to Quality Family Sleep

Sleep is an important component of our lives, yet it is often overlooked in our pursuit of a busy lifestyle. The need of enough sleep cannot be emphasized, as it is critical to our entire health and well-being. In this detailed book, we'll look at the science of sleep and give you practical tips on how to sleep better. Whether you're a busy professional, a health enthusiast, or a fitness novice, the advice in this post will help you get the rest you need.

Understanding the Fundamentals of Sleep

The Effects of Sleep on Health

7 Sleep Enhancement Strategies

Tip 1: Create a Consistent Sleep Schedule

Tip 2: Create the Ideal Sleep Environment

Tip 3: Include Physical Activity in Your Day

Tip 4: Nutrition and Sleep

Tip 5: Stress Management for Better Sleep

Tip 6: Digital Detoxification and Relaxation

Tip 7: Learn Relaxation Techniques

Bonus Tip 4

Tracking Your Sleep Progress

Quality sleep is more than just closing your eyes and falling asleep. It is a complex physiological process that has a significant impact on our overall health. To really appreciate the value of sleep, we must first comprehend its fundamental mechanics.

Sleep patterns: Sleep is made up of alternating cycles of REM (Rapid Eye Movement) and NREM (Non-Rapid Eye Movement) sleep, each with its own unique characteristics and functions. The significance of deep sleep: Deep NREM sleep is where physical repair and restoration take place, which benefits general health.

Dreaming and REM sleep: REM sleep is linked to vivid dreams and is essential for cognitive function, learning, and memory consolidation.

The Effects of Sleep on Health

Quality sleep is not a luxury; it is a must for optimum health. The advantages of getting enough sleep extend to many facets of your life.

Sleep is necessary for memory consolidation, problem solving, and decision making.

Physical health: Sleep promotes immune function and hormone regulation, which aids in muscle repair and growth.

Emotional health: Sleep deprivation can cause mood changes and increased stress, negatively impacting mental health.

7 Sleep Improvement Tips:

Tip 1: Create a Regular Sleep Schedule

A regular sleeping schedule is the cornerstone of excellent sleep. Here's how you can make one:

Every day, even on weekends, go to bed and wake up at the same hour.

This regimen assists in regulating your body's internal clock, making it simpler to sleep and wake up refreshed.

Tip 2: Create an Ideal Sleep Environment

Your sleeping environment has a significant impact on the quality of your sleep.

To make it ideal, make your bedroom dark, quiet, and chilly.

Purchasing a nice mattress and pillows.

To filter out undesired light, use blackout curtains.

Tip 3: Include Physical Activity in Your Daily Routine

Exercise on a regular basis can considerably improve your sleep. Consider the following suggestions:

Participate in aerobic exercises such as jogging, cycling, or swimming.

Each week, aim for at least 150 minutes of moderate-intensity exercise.

Vigorous workouts should be avoided close to bedtime because they can be stimulating.

Tip 4: Nutrition and Sleep

What and when you eat can have an impact on your sleep quality:

Before going to bed, avoid eating anything heavy or spicy.

Choose lighter, more balanced snacks.

Caffeine and alcohol use should be monitored, especially in the afternoon and evening.

Tip 5: Stress Management for Better Sleep

Stress and sleep are inextricably linked. To deal with stress, try the following methods:

Try practicing mindfulness meditation.

Create a regular pre-sleep relaxing program.

If the stress is unbearable, consult a therapist or counselor.

Tip 6: Digital Detoxification and Relaxation

Reducing screen usage before bedtime will help you sleep better:

Turn off all electronic gadgets at least one hour before going to bed.

Relax by doing things like reading a book.

Reduce the brightness of the lights to indicate to your body that it is time to relax.

Tip 7: Learn Relaxation Techniques

Relaxation techniques can help you relax your thoughts and prepare your body for sleep:

Deep breathing techniques should be practiced.

Physical stress can be relieved by progressive muscle relaxation.

Visualization exercises might assist you in shifting your focus away from stress.

Bonus Tips:

- Consider the following natural sleep remedies to improve your sleep quality:

- Relaxation can be aided by herbal drinks such as chamomile and valerian root.

- When diffused or applied topically, lavender essential oil may have a relaxing effect.

- A sleep mask might help you sleep better by blocking out undesirable light.

Tracking Your Sleep Progress

To track your progress, keep a sleep journal. If your sleep problems persist, seek advice from a healthcare practitioner. Sometimes underlying health issues can interfere with your sleep.

Conclusion

No matter how hectic your schedule is, you can get enough sleep. You may build a sleep-friendly schedule that improves your well-being by following these steps and recognizing the value of sleep. Remember that getting enough sleep leads to more productivity, better fitness gains, and a healthier you.

Creating a Restful Sleep Environment

Decluster Your Space

Before your body can begin to slumber, it is necessary to maintain your sleeping environment clean and free of any distractions. Unwanted job papers, cluttered artwork, or even a treadmill are all unpleasant reminders of your responsibilities that may keep you awake at night. Hoarding can have a negative impact on sleep in the worst-case situation.

Instead, make your bedroom clutter-free and your décor as simple as possible. It's also a good idea to get rid of any blue-light emitters, such as screen devices. These devices can be distracting even when turned off.

Utilize Essential Oils

We naturally correlate calming scents with emotions and memories, which influence how we feel. Essential oils for sleep are sometimes overlooked, despite the fact that they can help you wind down, relax, and eventually fall asleep throughout the night.

Aromatherapy smells made from essential oils are an easy and inexpensive approach to help you relax physically and mentally. Aromatherapy promotes a restful sleep environment. Lavender and vanilla are two of the most popular natural sleep oil smells. They can be vaporized or diffused in an aromatherapy diffuser.

Invest in a New Mattress

Examine your sleeping posture because this will determine if a soft or firm bed would help you sleep better. Whatever sort of mattress you prefer—memory foam, natural fiber, or a cooling and heating mattress—try it out in-store if possible.

Don't worry if you can't try a mattress before purchasing it. Mail order mattresses are also available with free home trials.

Some mattresses are designed with specific health conditions in mind, while generic pressure point mattresses can often aid with pain difficulties. If you have sleep apnea, sciatica, scoliosis, or another ailment, consult your doctor before shopping for a new mattress.

Although most mattresses last up to ten years, making the initial purchase can be intimidating. If money is tight, you can add foam toppers to your mattress to boost comfort and prevent you from waking up stiff and achy. Looking into better bedding when choosing a new mattress is also important for improving your sleep environment.

Set Your Bedroom's Temperature

The ideal sleeping temperature is around 65 degrees Fahrenheit (18.3 degrees Celsius). This varies from person to person, but most doctors recommend setting the thermostat between 60 and 67 degrees Fahrenheit (15.6 to 19.4 degrees Celsius) for the best sleep.

Choose a soothing color for your bedroom walls.

Color has a strong influence on our emotions and can help us sleep better by creating a calming environment. Blue is the greatest bedroom hue for sleeping, according to study, followed by yellow, green, and silver.

Blue light, on the other hand, can have the opposite impact. Adding blue light to your room does not improve it. Stick to neutral, pastel, or modest colors, as strong colors may trick the brain into thinking it needs to be alert.

Set your bed apart for sleeping only.

Only if you stop from working, watching TV, or using your phone, tablet, or computer will your brain begin to associate the bedroom with sleep. This will make it much easier for you to relax at night.

Keep the volume low.

Earplugs are one way to deal with distracting noises, and you can even consider soundproof tiles to keep noise out of your bedroom. If you are still having difficulty keeping things quiet, consider transferring your bedroom to another room whenever possible.

If you cannot prevent or remove noise generated by your neighbors, traffic, or other folks in your household, consider sleeping with a fan on to hide the sounds.

Consider Purchasing New Bedding

When shopping for the greatest sort of sheets, you will notice a vast range of thread counts, weaves, and materials. All of these factors contribute to the warmth and softness of the sheets, and the finest bed sheets for you should be dependent on how you wish to sleep.

Do you ever wake up shivering in the middle of the night despite having an abundance of clothing on? Fleece and wool are two of the most popular cold-weather clothing selections, followed by silk.

On the other hand, you might wake up thinking you were sleeping in a steam room. If this describes you, you should look at different bedding textiles including cotton, linen, or even bamboo bed sheets. Bed sheets with breathable fabric and temperature-regulating properties let you sleep through the night by holding less heat, making them excellent for "hot sleepers."

Enhance Your Lighting

The bedroom should be completely dark. If there is a lot of light coming in via the windows, room-darkening coverings or drapes can help. If you frequently wake up in the middle of the night to use the restroom, a small night light in the bedroom can assist you in safely exiting the room.

While LED lights use less energy, they emit more blue light. Using dim or red lights before bedtime may help you sleep better. Before going to bed, avoid direct exposure to bright light. This will help you keep your regular sleeping routine.

Furthermore, natural light during the day may be overlooked when it comes to getting a decent night's sleep. Nonetheless, it is one of the most important factors in assisting you to sleep properly.

Discover the Ideal Pillow for You

To maintain spinal alignment while sleeping, it is recommended that you replace your pillow every one to two years. If, on the other hand, you notice that you are unable to feel comfortable while awake, or if you wake up with headaches, neck issues, or shoulder pains, you should consider replacing your pillow as soon as possible.

Consider your sleeping position before deciding on the right level of firmness for your pillow, which can range from soft options like down pillows to firmer ones like buckwheat pillows. Most people who sleep on their stomachs prefer thinner pillows, while those who sleep on their backs prefer medium-support pillows. Larger pillows are preferred by those who sleep on their sides.

Furthermore, if you have allergies or asthma, you should consider utilizing hypoallergenic mattresses and pillows, which protect you from allergens that could activate your symptoms. More ideas can be found in our guidelines for better sleeping with asthma.

Before entering your bedroom, prepare yourself for better sleep.

Workplace stress, family obligations, and illness can all interfere with sleep. Quality sleep may appear to be elusive. You can't constantly deal with sleep-robbing situations. You can, however, adopt sleep-promoting activities. Follow these guidelines.

Maintain a Timetable

A healthy adult requires at least seven hours of sleep per night. Maintain the same sleep routine every night and morning, including weekends. The sleep-wake cycle is strengthened by consistency.

Try something calming if you haven't fallen asleep after 20 minutes. Relax by reading a book or making a simple craft. When you're tired, go back to bed and rest. Maintain a relatively steady sleep and wake-up schedule, but allow yourself to become nervous if you struggle to fall asleep one night.

Eat and drink with caution.

Don't go to bed hungry or full, but watch what you consume before bed. Large meals should be avoided two hours before bedtime. You may be kept awake by pain. Caffeinated beverages should also be avoided. If you consume coffee too late in the day, it can keep you awake for hours.

Relax

Cool, dark, and serene. Evening light may make it difficult to sleep. Avoid using bright displays before going to bed. Consider sleeping with room-darkening drapes, earplugs, a fan, or other objects that induce chilly, dark silence.

Bathing or other relaxation techniques before bedtime may help you sleep better. Try breathing exercises for sleep and relaxing with a book or a warm shower.

Daytime naps should be kept to a minimum.

Naps may interfere with nighttime sleep if they are too long or too late. Late-day naps should be limited to one hour. If you work at night, you may need to take a power nap before work to catch up on sleep.

Exercise on a daily basis

Sleep is improved by regular exercise. Simply avoid activity before bedtime and try to do it in the morning or afternoon if possible, or in the early evening if that's the ideal time for you. Maintaining a solid workout regimen requires consistency, and spending time outside every day may help with sleep by exposing you to natural light.

Control Your Anxiety and Stress

Address your worries before going to bed. Write down your thoughts for tomorrow so they don't bother you while you sleep. Begin by organizing, prioritizing, and delegating tasks.

Medication

While this ***should only be used as a last resort***, drugs may help you fall asleep faster, especially if you have a sleep condition. If you choose to utilize medicine to help you sleep better, it should be used sparingly and only after being medically examined and recommended by a doctor.

Questions and Answers

- Is the environment a factor in sleep?

Yes, your surroundings might influence how easy it is for you to fall and stay asleep. Too much light, noise, and being too hot or cold might make it difficult to relax enough to sleep. An uncomfortable mattress and bedding can also prevent you from falling asleep when it's time to sleep. Of course, there are other reasons you may not be sleeping well, such as sleep disorders, so if you are having difficulty sleeping, you should consult a sleep specialist.

- How can I keep noise out of my bedroom?

If earplugs aren't quiet enough for you, you can look at techniques to block noise from your bedroom. Heavy drapes and soundproofing tiles are quick ways to keep noise out, and larger doors and windows may be worth considering as well. If the sound appears to be coming from a certain wall or via a window, you may wish to move the bed or even change rooms.

- Can a cluttered room interfere with your sleep?

Yes, having a cluttered bedroom might make it difficult to fall asleep. When you close your eyes and see the clutter, you may begin to think about cleaning and other activities, making it difficult to relax and fall asleep.

- How can I make my bedroom a sleep sanctuary?

It's critical to keep distractions to a minimum when designing a bedroom for better sleep. Make the room as dark, chilly, and silent as possible. Clearing out electronic screen gadgets like tablets and computers can help you sleep better, but you don't have to adopt minimalism to have a good sleeping environment.

Relaxation is also essential. Some people find that having plants in their bedrooms helps them sleep better. Others may choose a comfort object, such as a plush animal or a pillow to cuddle.

- What is the most significant aspect of a bedroom?

Naturally, having one of the greatest mattresses is the most important aspect of getting a good night's sleep. If you can't settle down and become comfortable, you're unlikely to fall asleep quickly and may miss out on restorative sleep. However, you should not neglect the importance of having the correct pillows and bedding, as these can mean the difference between feeling nice, warm, and supported when sleeping.

Consider using any of these healthy sleep practices if you have difficulty falling or staying asleep or if you want to improve the quality of your sleep. If your sleeping problems persist, you should consult your primary care physician.

Chapter 5: Mental Wellness Magic

When you hear the words "mental wellness," you might think of a state of perpetual delight. But it goes beyond that. The human body, brain, and way of life must perform a complicated dance while accommodating a wide spectrum of emotions. Instead of being continuously cheerful, the key to mental wellness is navigating through these numerous life events and emotions with a sense of harmony.

Continue reading to learn what mental wellness is and how to achieve mental wellbeing in your own life.

What exactly is Mental Wellness?

According to the World Health Organization (WHO), mental wellbeing is "a state of well-being in which the individual realizes his or her own abilities, can cope with the normal stresses of life, can work productively and fruitfully, and is able to make a contribution to his or her community."

Take note of how this term makes no mention of happiness. It also does not imply the absence of mental disorder.

Rather, mental wellbeing involves being able to manage with the challenges of life, whether they are as basic as a work project or as complex as a breakup. It is the harmony of your emotional, bodily, spiritual, and mental selves.

How Can I Improve My Mental Health?

Not sure if you passed the mental health test? Having one or more of these symptoms on a regular basis could be an early warning indication of a larger problem:

- Excessive or insufficient eating or sleeping Distancing from people and customary activities

- Having little to no energy

- Feeling numb or as if nothing is important

- Experiencing unexplainable aches and pains

- Helpless or hopeless feelings

- Excessive smoking, drinking, or drug use

- Feeling particularly agitated, furious, upset, anxious, or terrified

- Fighting or yelling at family and friends

- Having significant mood swings

- Consider harming yourself or others.

- Inability to carry out daily responsibilities

If you or a loved one exhibits one or more of these signs, it may be time to turn your attention to improving your mental health. Improving mental wellbeing can look different for each person, but there are some general recommendations to follow if you want to work on it. **These are some examples:**

- Allowing oneself to seek professional assistance if necessary

- Keeping in touch with friends, family, and the community

- Finding ways to maintain a good attitude

- Including physical activity in your daily routine

- Volunteering and assisting others

- Developing the correct coping skills for you

How Can You Improve Your Mental Health?

The key to improving your mental health is to focus on one aspect of your life at a time. For example, one week can be dedicated to activities such as yoga, mindfulness, and meditation, which can help you live "in the moment." This entails letting go of past and future concerns and focusing solely on what is happening in the present moment.

The following week can be devoted to rest and leisure. While staying busy is great, make sure to take pauses and not be too hard on yourself. Burnout and poor coping techniques can result from a lack of relaxation, both physically and mentally.

Another week might be dedicated to spending quality time with family and friends. This is an excellent technique to improve mental wellness. A day spent with your best friend or family can help you cope with trauma, boost your self-esteem, and improve your mood.

5 Activities for Better Mental Health

There are certain activities you may engage in to improve your mental health and balance your mental, physical, spiritual, and emotional selves. To get you started, here are five examples:

1.   Feed your mind. When life gets chaotic, it's easy to put job, social life, or other priorities ahead of your own. However, your dietary health is critical. Determine which foods make you feel the best and stick to them.

2. Get your heart rate up. Exercise generates endorphins—the 'feel good' chemical—to flood your brain while also decreasing   cortisol—the stress chemical. Aim for at least 15 minutes of activity per day.

3. Create and stick to a sleeping regimen. The average adult needs seven (7)-nine (9) hours of sleep every night. If you have difficulty sleeping, creating morning and nighttime routines around sleep, such as stretching, writing,

showering, reading, or any activity that helps you wind down at night and get up in the morning, may be beneficial.

4. Do something at which you excel. Are you a fantastic painter? Are you a focused musician? Are you a fast runner? Get that adrenaline rush that comes with knowing what you're doing and doing it well. Don't know what your strengths are yet? That's even better. Explore several hobbies and interests until you find something that interests you.

5. When you need assistance, ask for it. You are not alone in your difficulties, no matter how big or small. Don't feel obligated to be strong and push through your problems; instead, make sure you have a solid support network or a healthcare expert to speak it out with.

Overall Wellness Requires Mental Wellness

While there is no one-size-fits-all solution or magic formula for mental health and wellness, there are numerous tools and tactics at your disposal. Not all of them will work for you, but experimenting with different strategies will help you discover your own secret formula for success. If at first you don't succeed, try, try again, as the old adage goes.

Stress-Busting Strategies for the Whole Family

Stress is an inevitable aspect of life. We all experience stress in a variety of conditions, forms, and levels. What creates stress for one person may appear less to another. Stress can be caused by seemingly minor events such as heavy traffic or a long line at the store, or it can be caused by a crisis event such as the loss of a job, the death of a family member, a pandemic such as that caused by the novel coronavirus, the virus that causes the infectious disease COVID-19, or the catastrophic flooding experienced in mid-Michigan.

To avoid unpleasant physical and mental repercussions, the most crucial thing to do is to acknowledge, understand, and manage your stress. Unmanaged stress can develop into chronic stress. Chronic stress has been found to weaken the immune system, raise blood pressure and sugar levels, and aggravate underlying illnesses such as anxiety and depression.

It might take some time to figure out which stress management strategies work best for you. While there is no ideal method to deal with stress, here are some suggestions that may help you and your family:

Understand your own stress signals. For example, do you get forgetful, short-tempered, clumsy, or something else when you are stressed? Consider what draws your attention the most. Examine your children and other family members for symptoms of stress and request that they do the same for you. Other individuals may detect our stress signs before we do.

Make time to do something significant, soothing, and enjoyable for you and your family. Read a book, relax on the porch and take in the view, have coffee with a friend, or have a movie or game night with the family.

Deep breathing or mindfulness exercises are recommended. When you begin to feel worried and tense, try sitting and breathing for a minute or two. It helps to mentally repeat, "I am breathing in, and I am breathing out." It may appear stupid, but it keeps your mind on something you can control: your breath. It helps to calm your thoughts and relax you. Teach children how to utilize their breath to relax. Include family breathing pauses in your regular activities. The more you practice this while you are not anxious, the simpler it will be to access when you are stressed.

Get adequate rest. Most health professionals agree that people who receive at least 8 hours of sleep every night are less worried, depressed, and able to regulate their anger. If feasible, take an afternoon nap to complement your sleep demands. Even a 15-minute "cat nap" might be incredibly relaxing for some individuals. Just try not to snooze away the day so you can sleep at night. Maintain a healthy sleep routine for your children as well.

Accept your sensations and emotions. It is OK to be unhappy, nervous, furious, or stressed. Noticing and acknowledging these feelings might help us be more sympathetic to ourselves. Convince yourself like you would a best friend: "Wow, I'm sorry to hear you're stressed/anxious. I am here to help you. "Do you need a hug?" Recognizing and naming your children's tense or nervous emotions, followed by a hug, might help them accept them.

Consider your family members' emotional requirements. In a crisis, our priorities may alter abruptly. During the rehabilitation process, make sure you understand and respect the requirements of family members or other home inhabitants. Adults must model proper emotional reactions for children, according to North Dakota State University Extension, since keeping balance and serenity will help them negotiate their own emotions.

Save your energy on things you can influence. There are several events over which we have no control. Instead of focusing on what-if situations, focus on activities and actions that you can perform to start the process of restoration, healing, or returning to normal.

Create or utilize a support system. Your support system is made up of people who may or may not play diverse roles in your life. Make use of your support system to talk about your feelings and get help. If you are unable to socialize in person, reach out to individuals via social media, text messaging, email, or video chats to feel more connected to your support network. You may also be making them feel more connected.

Laughter is the most effective medication. Laughter and humor are excellent stress relievers and enhance well-being. Look for some family-friendly humor. Hold a family joke-telling competition.

Concentrate on your own health as well as the health of individuals in your household. Individuals will frequently turn to alcohol and drugs as a coping method during difficult situations. These actions can lead to increased tension and anxiety. Instead, focus on good habits like eating more fruits and vegetables and drinking more water. Aim for at least 30 minutes of physical activity every day. You may accomplish this by going for a stroll around the house or neighborhood, or by playing music and dancing. You could even hold a family dancing contest in which everyone teaches each other a new dance move.

Seek expert assistance. If you are feeling overwhelmed, get help from a specialist, such as your primary care physician or a mental health expert.

Cultivating Resilience and Emotional Well-being

Our mental health has never been more important in today's fast-paced and demanding world. Mental health is more than just problems. It serves as a reminder of the global need for and relevance of mental health awareness. Emotional, cognitive, psychological, and social well-being are all components of mental health. It determines how one handles stress, makes decisions, and acts in daily life. The difficulties we confront in our personal and professional lives can have a negative impact on our ability to thrive and find joy.

Mental health issues can affect anyone. Sometimes an unforeseen impediment can appear in one's path, leaving them stressed and unsure of what to do. And, on some days, nothing; no motivation, no inventiveness. And then one becomes tortured by self-doubt. A person's mental wellness does not guarantee that they will never face difficulties, disappointments, or loss. People with good mental health recover more quickly from trauma and stress.

We've been taught that it's 'acceptable' to ignore the emotional signals that tell us something is wrong and try to cope by distracting ourselves. According to an

HBR survey, 61% of employees are burned out and are increasingly seeking mental health care. According to a WHO assessment, anxiety and despair increased by more than 25% during the first year of the pandemic. While this statistic increased fast, therapy for mental health disorders did not. In fact, it was understaffed.

While individuals suffering from mental health concerns may frequently feel confined, businesses can have a huge positive impact. Many organizations have now prioritized mental health programs and are addressing this issue by devising techniques to reduce the stigma associated with the state of not being okay. Organizations are going to great lengths to help their employees on their mental health journey, from monthly mental health days off to weekly yoga and meditation sessions. Employees are encouraged to take a break from their regular routine and relax their minds and bodies.

Nevertheless, many people suffer from mental health problems because they either have inertia while beginning any mental workout or simply do not have time to devote to meditation or other activities. It is past time to acknowledge the critical relevance of addressing mental health as a means of unlocking resilience and flourishing in the face of hardship. We can pave the road for a brighter and more satisfying future by accepting this paradigm change. The following are some helpful strategies for practicing mindfulness and making it a part of one's life in order to improve one's mental health.

Perspective Shifts: Priority Given to Mental Health

Mental health is not an afterthought or a luxury; it is the foundation of our complete well-being. It includes our emotional, psychological, and social well-being, and it influences how we think, feel, and act in all aspects of our life. We empower ourselves to address mental health with the same urgency and importance as physical health by acknowledging its basic role.

Meditation can help you practice mindfulness.

Meditation promotes inner calm by increasing awareness of one's thoughts, emotions, mental barriers, prejudices, and thought patterns. Meditation does not have to be a difficult task; it can be as simple as 10 minutes of focused breathing per day.

Concentrate on the method rather than the goals.

To improve one's mental health, it is common to set a month-long goal of attaining a state of mindfulness. However, such objectives undermine the purpose of mindfulness. To be at peace, one must concentrate on and adhere to a system. Instead of saying, "I will cure my mental illness in one month," instead, "I will meditate for 15 minutes every day." Once the system is in place, the results begin to appear automatically.

Be kind with yourself.

It is natural for the mind to wander during one's first steps toward awareness. Instead of becoming frustrated, condemning oneself, or obsessing over a single thought, one should be gentle to oneself and recognize how difficult it is to detach from one's thoughts and surroundings.

Prioritizing mental health is a necessity in today's difficult society, not an indulgence. We lay the groundwork for personal and communal growth by supporting mental health. While employers nowadays are hyper-vigilant in addressing mental health difficulties at work, individuals should also recognize that it is acceptable to take a mental health break or leave a setting in which they do not feel comfortable. There are numerous strategies to reduce stress, whether you wish to manage a specific mental health problem, handle emotions better, or simply feel more cheerful. Feeling one's emotions does not make one weak or negative; rather, it makes one more authentic to oneself. Let us work together to prioritize mental health and create a more resilient, vibrant, and compassionate world.

Chapter 6: Holistic Health at Home

Holistic health considers the full individual in terms of health and healing, including the body, mind, and spirit, as well as the environmental aspects of daily life. A holistic approach emphasizes the fact that the whole is made up of many interconnected pieces. When one component of the individual is out of balance or neglected, it affects the other parts.Holistic health places the majority of one's health in the hands of the individual, through thoughtful and educated decisions, self-study, education, and a natural way of living. Holistic health practitioners and approaches are designed to assist individuals in living a whole-person healthy lifestyle.

Personal choice, observation, and commitment are required for health and healing—learning to tune into your experience and understand what works, what exacerbates symptoms, and what nourishes your entire being.

Learning the fundamentals of holistic health may help you navigate your health and healing journey with awareness and inspiration to aid you along the way.

Continue reading for an introduction to holistic health.

The Advantages of Holistic Health

There are numerous advantages of incorporating holistic health practices into your daily life:

Treatment of the common cold

Reducing inflammation in the body Reducing daily stress Adding medications, meals, or daily habits that are beneficial additions to feeling your best

Zinc and elderberry, for example, two natural therapies, have been demonstrated to reduce the duration of the common cold. Turmeric, a well-known root, has been demonstrated to reduce systemic inflammation and arthritic symptoms in patients. Acupuncture has been demonstrated to be an effective pain therapy. Aromatherapy has been demonstrated to promote healthy sleep and minimize anxiety in patients undergoing cardiac stent implantation in an intensive care unit.

There are numerous holistic health therapies and regimens available from various traditions around the world. Finding a modality that works for you and that is compatible with any other medical therapy or medication you are receiving is certainly worthwhile.

Many people prefer to supplement more conventional treatments with holistic living techniques, which is known as supplementary or integrative medicine. Some of the more ancient holistic health approaches have even been adopted into regular medical care in several circumstances.

Some holistic health methods require a trained practitioner, while others, such as meditation or yoga, can be self-taught mind-body activities to explore on your own.

Here are a few holistic healthcare options for you to consider.

Functional Medicine

Functional medicine is a science-based approach to identifying and treating the underlying cause of disease. Each symptom and diagnosis could be one of several variables influencing an individual's overall health and fitness.

To define and prioritize a treatment plan, functional medicine practitioners frequently assemble scientific tests, such as blood work. Working with a functional medicine practitioner will frequently include dietary and lifestyle recommendations such as healthy eating, professional supplement regimens, sleep support, stress management, exercise protocols, hormonal health strategies, and mind-body practices.For example, one 28-week trial examined a functional medicine approach to relieving stress, energy, fatigue, digestive disorders, and quality of life in middle-aged women. The study found that stress, exhaustion, and quality-of-life capacities improved. According to this study, functional medicine offers a potent and practical solution to a wide range of health issues, from stress management to gastrointestinal pain.

Ayurveda

Ayurveda is an ancient Indian medicine that is regarded to be one of the world's oldest treatments. Ayurveda has evolved over thousands of years and is currently practiced in countries all over the world. Ayurveda is a supplemental medicine that examines the whole individual through several health perspectives.

Ayurveda is well-known for its capacity to heal a wide range of diseases, including cancer, diabetes, arthritis, and asthma. Ayurveda is a holistic medical approach that addresses physical, psychological, philosophical, ethical, and spiritual well-being. Ayurveda promotes various aspects of the body's self-healing abilities through a body, mind, and soul approach, as well as the use of herbal remedies to treat specific disorders and conditions.

While more research is needed to scientifically validate many parts of Ayurveda as a holistic therapeutic strategy, significant progress has been made in developing a deeper knowledge of how Ayurveda works and its effectiveness with many of today's most common health conditions.

Acupuncture

Acupuncture started and was used in China more than 3,000 years ago as part of traditional Chinese medicine. Acupuncture is built on a complex network of meridians, which are energy highways in the body through which qi (or energy) should flow. The meridians are frequently described as passageways or channels that run throughout the body, providing access to various systems and transporting blood and physiological fluids.

"Although the meridians have not been reliably identified as actual anatomical structures, they appear to serve as a road map to identify the location of various acupoints," according to one study. Acupoints, according to research, overlie important neural bundles."

Acupuncture generally employs needles, suction cups, and pressure points at specific meridians on the body to activate and strengthen the meridians, resulting in increased health and energy. While more research is needed, there has been a lot of good news about acupuncture being an effective treatment for specific health concerns like pain and headaches.

Nutritional Therapy

Nutritional medicine is a holistic health approach that stresses the role of diet and nutrition in overall health and wellness. As Hippocrates famously said, "Let food be thy medicine, and medicine be thy food," nutritional therapies stress food as medicine.

Nutritional medicine practitioners also look specifically at the individual and design an eating plan to match exactly what is uniquely suited to the patient's current health status and bio-individuality—the patient's unique and specific nutritional needs based on a variety of important factors and variables such as climate, genetic lineage, environmental stressors, and daily life rhythms.

Food is essential to an individual's health, according to rising research in this sector. Notably, diet is a low-cost method and supplement to the prevention and treatment of many common health problems, including diabetes and many of its associated disorders (weight gain, high cholesterol, and high blood pressure).

Chiropractic

When a chiropractor performs spinal manipulation, commonly known as a chiropractic adjustment, it is the most well-known chiropractic treatment. A chiropractor will most commonly utilize joint manipulation, soft tissue manipulation, physical rehabilitation or home care, and activity assistance to reduce pain and inflammation, improve nerve function, and/or release built-up pressure on joints.

Chiropractic can be daunting at first because physical adjustments involve a level of vulnerability, but a good chiropractic adjustment can feel like a huge relief. According to research, the most prevalent reasons for seeking chiropractic care are low back pain, neck discomfort, and extremities issues. Other elements of health, such as diet, vitamins, home movement therapies, and stress management, are frequently addressed by chiropractors.

Aromatherapy

Aromatherapy (also known as essential oil treatment) is a holistic health method that promotes health and well-being by using natural plant extracts in the form of oils. Aromatherapy is the medical application of a wide range of aromatic essential oils (topically, internally, and aromatically) to promote body, mind, and spirit health. Aromatherapy has been shown to improve both physical and mental wellbeing.

Oregano oil, for example, is frequently used internally to increase immunity, whilst chamomile oil is used topically to decrease stress. There are numerous plant-based essential oils to investigate and match with various areas of your health and well-being.

Meditation

You can create a deep state of inner peace that affects many areas of your being just by sitting quietly, slowing your breath, and developing a one-pointed focus such as a mantra or an affirmation.

Meditation is a holistic health practice that you may do on your own, in the comfort of your own home, and on your own schedule once you understand the basics.

Meditation comes in numerous forms and styles, including spiritual, internal or externally focused, and progressive muscle relaxation, and it originated in a range of cultures around the world. Finding a style that suits your requirements is a smart place to begin.

While additional study is needed, several studies have found that meditation is an excellent technique to engage in a mind-body approach to healing. According to research, meditation can help with health issues like excessive blood pressure, cardiovascular health, and inflammation.Many novices choose guided meditation at first to learn the fundamentals and become acquainted with meditation. You might also look for a meditation teacher or group in your area or online.

Yoga

Yoga is a collection of physical, mental, and spiritual activities that originated 3,000 years ago in ancient India. Yoga emphasizes the mind-body connection through deliberate movement and postures (asana), as well as breathwork and focused attention. Yoga can also have a scholarly component, such as the well-known literature The Yoga Sutras, which describes the philosophy of yoga and was initially translated from one of India's well-known sages, Patanjali.

Numerous studies have proved that yoga may be used to prevent and treat many of today's most common health conditions, including blood glucose levels, musculoskeletal diseases, and a healthy cardiovascular system. Yoga has also been shown to benefit health by lowering anxiety, promoting good emotions, and improving mental focus.

If you are new to yoga, start slowly and learn the fundamentals so that you may develop on them over time. To get you started, most yoga studios offer beginner or foundation classes.

Holistic Health's Safety and Effectiveness

Few alternative remedies have been thoroughly explored and investigated. While holistic health therapies are generally safe and beneficial, you should conduct your own research. One method to reduce the hazards of holistic health is to consult with your health care practitioner before incorporating such treatments into your health regimen. Herbal and nutritional supplements, in particular, can be potent and can mix with pharmaceuticals or other natural therapies.

DIY Wellness for Every Family Member

It's no secret that our entire family has spent more time than ever before sitting in front of a screen somewhile ago due to the COVID 19 Pandemic. We could all win an Olympic couch surfing competition thanks to online school, regular Zoom meetings, and a lack of organized sports. We felt the draw of the couch and understood that, for our small family, getting some exercise makes us all better people. We also don't characterize the necessity for movement in terms of "getting a beach body." We discuss the mental and physical benefits of leading an active lifestyle.

We have a family rule that our children do not have to be professional athletes, but they must be active on most days. This does not imply that they must run a marathon, but they must get moving. Us too!

When it comes to your family's health, you truly need to work together. Create a family wellness plan to provide direction for everyone in your home.

Step one: Take into account everyone's goals, needs, and interests.

Every member of your family is unique, and those distinctions must be taken into account. Sit down and prepare a list for each person, including their age, dietary restrictions, health issues, and obligations. Consider the habits and routines that have developed in your home. Identifying what everyone requires to keep healthy will assist you in determining the best path to their specific goals.

Step two is to create a budget.

Looking at your family's demands and habits, it's possible that you all need more physical activity. Perhaps everyone has become too accustomed to that meal delivery service that delivers tacos and cupcakes in under 30 minutes (guilty). Examining your food and activity expenses can help you create a budget that permits you to join an online wellness program or a healthy food subscription service. Take into account all of your necessary spending when creating a budget to identify where you can make room and establish some new restrictions.

Step 3: Make a weekly schedule.

Schedules and lists are my drug of choice. They also keep me sane. Set a weekly family routine for grocery shopping, cooking, and physical activity. Teaching your children a nutritious dish or demonstrating the value of regular exercise will prepare them for a lifetime of better habits.

Here's an illustration:

Every Sunday, go grocery shopping and to the farmer's market. Prepare quick breakfast and lunch choices for the week.

Monday through Thursday: Everyone logs one hour of physical activity. It's their decision.

Monday through Friday: Everyone takes turns cooking dinner on their assigned night. Yes, it's messy when the kids take over, but I keep telling myself, "They're developing life skills" as they use every dish in the kitchen to prepare tacos.

Every Saturday, there is a family activity. Something physical, such as trekking or playing basketball.

Every week isn't ideal, but it's a solid starting point.

Step four: Choose your rewards.

A long-term objective for the entire family to work toward is an excellent approach to keep everyone on track; just be careful how you convey it to children. We all have the right to eat and sleep, thus words count. As an alternative to saying, "Let's eat healthy all week and on Friday nights we get pizza!" go with "If we meet our goal to cook dinner five nights this week we get to order in on the weekend." Yes, there's a good possibility they'll choose the pizza (who wouldn't?). When it comes to physical goals, the reward could be a hiking weekend or a sporting event, or it could be new workout gear or equipment if the budget allows.

Step five: Keep track of your progress.

Meet once a month to discuss how everyone is doing. What are our emotions like? What are our sleeping habits? How are things doing at work and school? Is it true that we all despise dancing cardio? (Is it just Penn?) As children grow older and schedules become more complicated, their needs and ambitions will shift. We must be adaptable. However, knowing where everyone is with their health is always vital so that you can make changes and remain on top of any

difficulties. It never hurts to be encouraged on a regular basis.

CHAPTER 7: Tech Tools for Health

Digital health, often known as digital healthcare, is a wide, multidisciplinary term that encompasses ideas from the convergence of technology and healthcare. Digital health is the application of digital transformation to the field of healthcare, encompassing software, hardware, and services. Mobile health (mHealth) apps, electronic health records (EHRs), electronic medical records (EMRs), wearable devices, telehealth and telemedicine, and personalized medicine are all included under the digital health umbrella.

Patients, practitioners, researchers, application developers, and medical device manufacturers and distributors are among the stakeholders in the digital health field. Today, digital healthcare is playing an increasingly significant role in healthcare.

The Latest Apps and Gadgets for Family Fitness

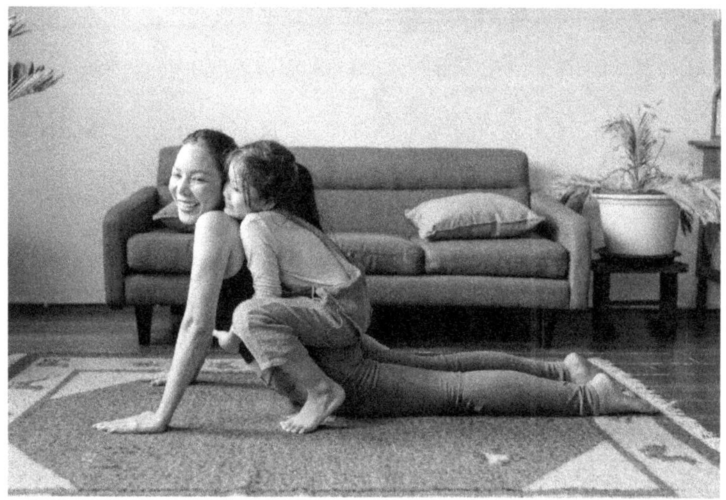

Working out and staying healthy has been a challenge over the previous year.

Working out has never been more entertaining, even if you're confined at home, thanks to updated gadgets and cutting-edge technologies on the market. It's time to wave goodbye to your couch potato alter ego and welcome to a better, healthier you.

Here are our top workout tools for transforming yourself into a fitness freak at home.

Intelligent Rope

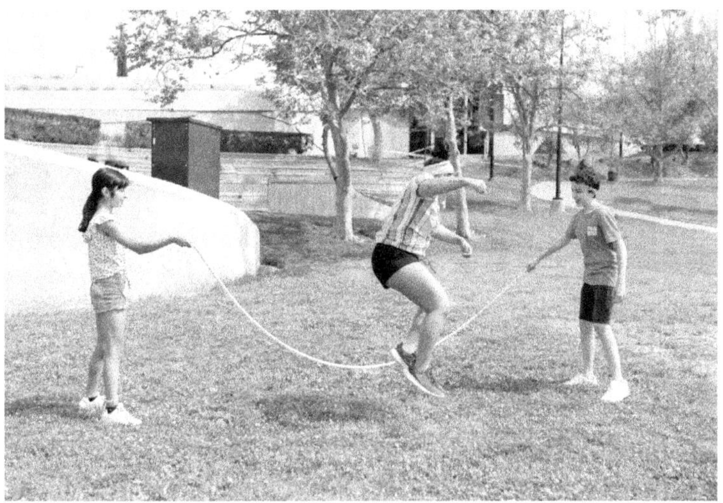

Using a skipping rope is one of the best cardio workouts you can do, and a smart rope may help you take it to the next level. A smart rope displays your fitness level in mid-air and assists you in storing workout data that is linked to your smartphone.

Wearable Technology

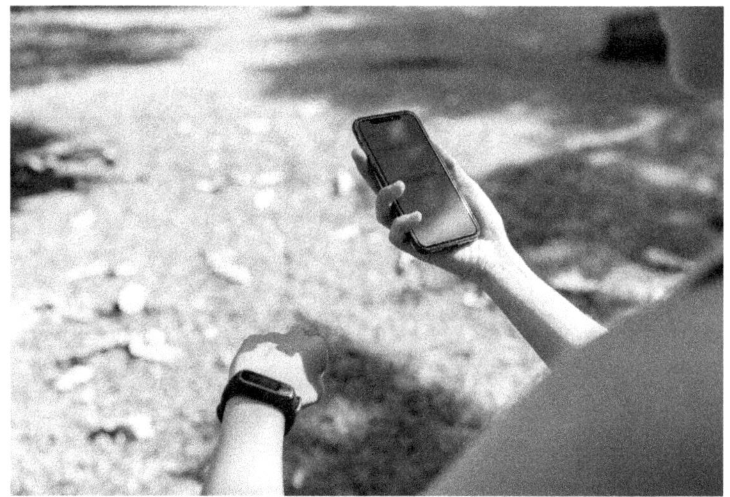

A smart watch is the ideal method to keep track of all your daily workouts and step counts. It connects the device to your phone and sends your progress and completed workout goals. It can also track your heart rate, steps, and oxygen levels.

Smart Workout Cycle

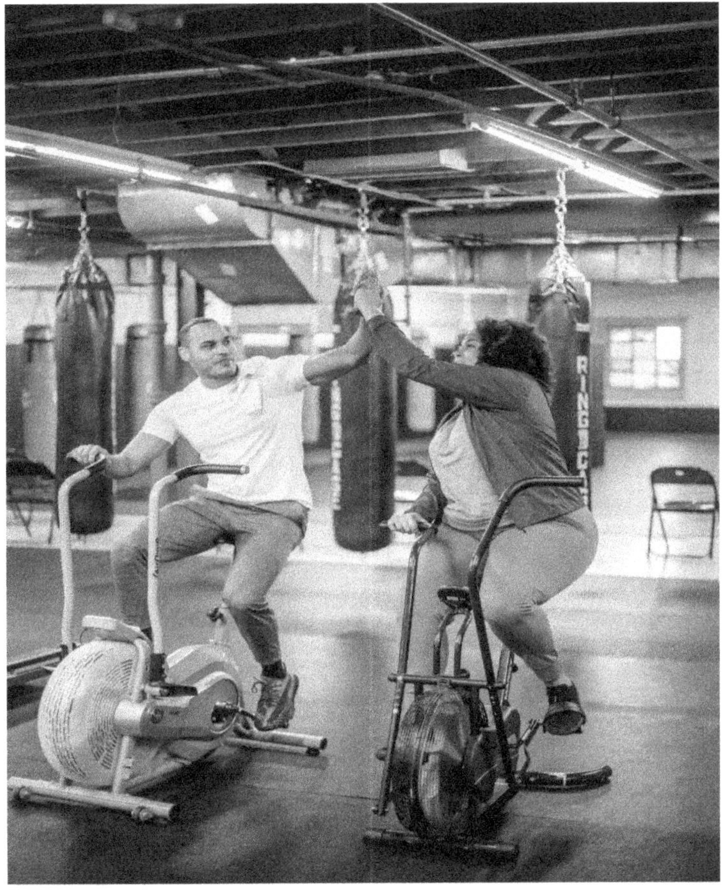

Do you miss going on an early morning bike ride with your fitness buddies?

We've got your back! A smart workout cycle is ideal for someone who enjoys being outside. It gives you the sensation of cycling through the empty streets of

your hometown.

Treadmill on Wheels

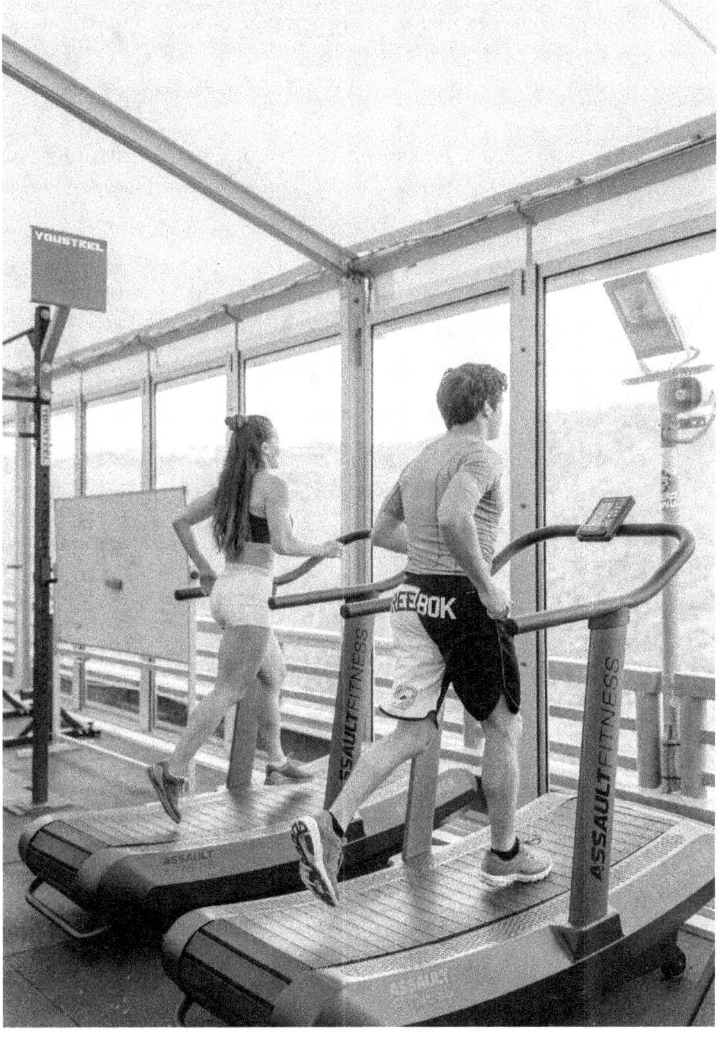

If you enjoy using the treadmill but find the cost excessive, not to mention the enormous amount of space it requires, this is the ideal workout gear for you. A portable treadmill is simple to operate and store. You can even intensify your workout while binge watching your favorite TV show.

Kettlebell with Intelligence

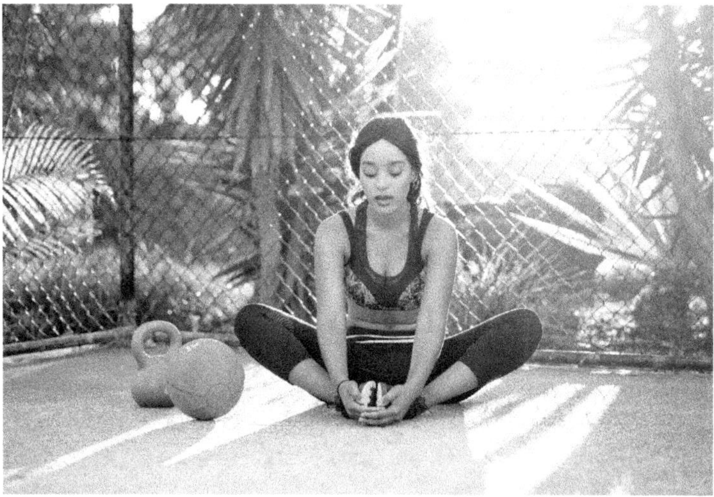

Too many kettlebells ruin the game? What if there was a single kettlebell that could replace all of the different weights you need? That is exactly what a smart kettlebell accomplishes. The weight of the bell may be adjusted to your specifications using the associated smartphone app, which can help you alter your strength exercises.

Balancing Screen Time and Well-being

In our digital age, screens have become an indispensable part of our lives. We are always surrounded by displays, whether on our smartphones, laptops, tablets, or televisions. While there is no doubt that technology has changed the way we work, live, and communicate, it is critical to understand the effects of excessive screen time on our health and wellness.

Prolonged screen use can disrupt sleep cycles, resulting in shorter sleep lengths and lower sleep quality, all of which can have a negative impact on our overall health.

In terms of mental health, excessive screen usage has been linked to elevated levels of stress, anxiety, and depression. Constant exposure to social media platforms can lead to feelings of inadequacy as we compare ourselves to meticulously manicured online portrayals of other people's lives. Screens and social media's addictive features can also lead to decreased productivity, a shorter attention span, and a sense of estrangement from the present. To enhance digital health, it is critical to build conscious technology use behaviors.

Here are some key ideas for balancing screen time and well-being:

Establish device-free zones: Screens should be forbidden at specific hours or in particular areas of your home. Make the bedroom, for example, a device-free zone to encourage improved sleep hygiene and relaxation.

Participate in frequent physical activities: As an alternative to screen time, promote physical activity and outdoor activities. Regular exercise not only benefits physical health but also aids in stress reduction, mood enhancement, and cognitive performance.

Practice digital detoxification: Take frequent breaks from screens, especially if you are using them for an extended amount of time. Consider setting out screen-free hours or even days to unplug from digital gadgets and engage in activities that promote relaxation and self-reflection.

Apply the 20-20-20 rule: Follow the 20-20-20 rule to prevent eye strain and promote eye health. Take a 20-second break every 20 minutes and fix your gaze on an item at least 20 feet away. This aids in the prevention of digital eye strain and the maintenance of good vision.

Encourage conscious technology use: Consider how and why you use screens. Establish specific goals for your screen usage and avoid mindless scrolling. Engage in things that nurture your well-being and practice being completely present in your interactions.

Adopting mindful technology use not only allows us to capitalize on technology's benefits for learning, productivity, and connectivity, but it also helps to mitigate any potential negative implications of excessive screen time. In the end, it is up to us to exercise control over our screen usage and prioritize our well-being in this technological age.

Chapter 8: Family Adventures in Wellness

There's no reason why spending time as a family needs to be costly. Family wellness is something that comes at no cost - and it can significantly improve your overall health! It all relies on what you do and how you go about doing it.

We put up this list of family wellness activities that will bring you and your loved ones closer together while also enhancing your health in a variety of vital ways.

One of our favorite family wellness recommendations is to go to the playground. If you have children, this is a terrific way to keep them active while still having fun! Playgrounds serve as a natural obstacle course, and you can get in a quick workout by pushing your kids on the swings or climbing on the jungle gym with them.

Some people believe that the ideal family wellness training takes place outside. That is why we are such great fans of nature walks. Nature walks are a terrific opportunity for families to spend time together while enjoying the fresh air that everyone requires for good mental and physical health. You can also do this activity elsewhere, such as on your sidewalk or on a nature trail in your town. This will also instill in your children a love of being outside, which is critical for their growth.

Everyone enjoys the water, and a pool or lake is a terrific place to have fun while simultaneously learning about swimming safety. Swimming is a crucial survival skill for both children and adults. You can enroll your children in swimming classes while also swimming in the pool, allowing you to spend time together while learning something new and remaining active.

Family Health and Wellness Activities

The list of family health and wellness activities is extensive. And it's fair that, after a long work week, preparing ahead for physical and mental well-being activities might seem like a hassle - but with a little additional effort, you can choose weekend activities that actually contribute to your energy levels rather than sap them).

To prevent wasting time over the weekend, all you have to do is spend some time planning an activity for the entire family so that everyone feels revived come

Monday and you can all share a bonding moment. Kids' health and wellness are more vital than ever, especially with so much of their time spent online, so don't neglect these wellness activities for kids!

We're sure you've never considered it, but getting enough sleep counts as a wellness activity. It is, in fact, one of the finest wellness activities for college students, as well as one of the best wellness activities for primary children. Everyone, regardless of age, might benefit from more sleep.

Meditation is another excellent health and wellness activity for children - and the entire family. Mindfulness has numerous advantages for children and teenagers; it can change the structure and function of the brain, improving the quality of thought and sensation. It can also improve self-esteem, tranquility, emotional intelligence, and sleep quality, as well as reduce anxieties and anxiety. Many schools have joined in, seeing this as one of the best health and wellness activities for pupils.

One of the most beneficial health and wellness activities for elementary pupils is art therapy. Instead of encouraging your child to unwind in front of a screen (which has been one of the most appealing COVID health activities for students), urge them to unwind through a creative activity. For decades, art therapy has been utilized to heal patients suffering from ailments ranging from stress to cancer.

Products for Family Wellness

Family wellness entails more than just what you do; it also includes what you have in your home. This collection of family wellness products includes everything from cold packs to vitamins.

Apart from vitamins, we recommend the following family wellness goods for your home:

Nasal spray is always a good idea. It aids in the relief of stuffy noses and allergy symptoms in both children and adults! It's a miracle remedy for stuffy noses, and you won't believe how quickly it works.

In a pinch, ear thermometers are also extremely useful. You may believe that you do not require a thermometer at home, but you will come to regret that decision when you need one the most and there is none to be found in your cupboards.

All Good Goop's all-natural healing balm works wonderfully for practically anything - if someone in your family gets a tiny scrape, burn, or bump, this is the product to use. It's even effective on diaper rash and chapped lips! This is useful in a pinch because no one wants to suffer through the discomfort associated with the ailments that this Goop can treat.

At-Home Wellness Activities

Wellness doesn't have to happen only on vacation or at the spa; there are many ways to include wellness activities into your daily routine. With these health activities at home, you may focus on your physical and emotional well-being without ever leaving your home (4).

Many individuals overlook the benefits of yoga. Yoga is ideal if you wish to improve your concentration and focus, boost your physiological awareness, and relieve tension. It's also a terrific physical activity for students to undertake at home - no extra equipment is required! Yoga has been demonstrated to raise GABA levels in the brain (a substance that helps to regulate nerve activity) and reduce anxiety symptoms.

Hiking is a popular choice among the many wellness activities for people at home. Getting outside for a short (or long) hike can reduce tension, anxiety, blood pressure, and cortisol levels - all of which have the ability to provide you with a relaxing impact that only nature can provide.

Bike riding is also a terrific way to improve your health! It can also help to relieve anxiety and stress from daily living, and it has the ability to boost memory, promote creative thinking, help you sleep better, and lower your risk of depression. Breathing in fresh air and keeping your legs moving can benefit not only your physical but also your mental health!

Wellness Activities and Games

Staying active is an excellent strategy to prevent chronic illnesses such as diabetes and hypertension, but health games and activities are also enjoyable (5)!

These enjoyable family activities are especially beneficial if you are bored with routine workouts.

Playing basketball is a terrific way to get your heart rate up and build camaraderie with your teammates. You may do this sport in your backyard or at the gym, and if you don't have a hoop, you can get creative and use a bucket.

Soccer is another wellness activity that you may be familiar with as one of the most enjoyable health class exercises. This game can be put up practically anywhere there is adequate space, and it is fun for the whole family to play. The best part is that while you're working to improve your game, you're also getting a full-body workout!

Another good choice is hula hooping, which is much more difficult than it appears. It doesn't take much equipment - just a hula hoop. Beyond that, all you need is enough space to get started. You may benefit from spinning the hula hoop by burning calories, burning fat, boosting cardiovascular health, and increasing your general balance.

Exemplifications of Healthy Physical Activity

Physical activity is an important aspect of being healthy, and it has numerous health advantages. You might be amazed at how many different sorts of physical activity you can undertake at home (6). You don't even have to leave the house to get your prescribed 150 minutes of exercise every week!

One of the first instances of everyday physical activity is as easy as stretching! Stretching simply includes utilizing your own body weight as a source of resistance, and it can improve circulation and lessen arthritis pain and inflammation. Stretching is one of the best examples of physical activity for seniors because of this.

Jumping rope is a fun healthy physical activity that we've been doing since we were children. You can do this inside or outside at any moment. You only need a jump rope. Jumping rope for a few minutes can increase your heart and lung fitness, bone strength, and balance and flexibility.

If you're seeking unusual examples of physical activity at home, here's one: Gardening. You're doing something good for your health if you have a green thumb and enjoy spending time in the garden. When you dig, mow the lawn, and weed, you're putting your body through a variety of movements and stretches that engage a wide range of muscles. Furthermore, you're spending precious time outside in the fresh air, which can significantly improve your mental health.

Making fitness a Family Affair

Children learn by example: if you read, they will read; if you consume healthy foods, they will eat nutritious foods; and if you exercise consistently, they will exercise routinely. Or, even better, why not get everyone involved in physical fitness activities together? The secret to a successful family exercise program is to keep things simple and enjoyable for everyone. Make your activities a family tradition that everyone enjoys.

Even moderate physical activity (along with a balanced diet) can help prevent your family members from heart disease, type 2 diabetes, and several types of cancer. Physical fitness activities are a fantastic method to release stress (i.e., fewer sibling conflicts) and send oxygen to the brain, so exercising on a regular basis could help keep the peace at home and increase academic achievement.

Before you begin your newfound fitness commitment, be sure that everyone in your family has received approval from your family doctor. To avoid muscle strain and injury, always increase your physical activity gradually. Stretch frequently and consume plenty of water.

CONCLUSION

Hey there, as we finish this journey together, let's savor the successes and look forward to new adventures in "Celebrating Achievements and Looking Forward."

This is a chapter of Your Family's Roadmap to a Healthier Future, not the end of a book.

Take a moment to celebrate your victories, whether it's completing a fitness challenge, establishing a new healthy routine, or simply having a good laugh over a nutritious meal. These triumphs are stepping stones on your family's individual journey to happiness.

And now, in "Looking Forward," see the road ahead as a continuation of your family's journey, rather than a dead end. What are you eager to tackle next? What goals do you have in mind? The future is a blank canvas ready for your family to paint it brightly.

Consider this book to be more than simply words; consider it to be Your Family's Roadmap to a Healthier Future. The comfortable times, shared delights, and devotion to well-being do not go with the last page. They are the beating hearts of your continuing family saga.

Allow this book to be a companion, a source of inspiration, and a reminder that your family's journey is ongoing as you shut it. Here's to Your Family's Healthier Future Roadmap—may the journey be filled with joy, accomplishments, and limitless experiences. Cheers to the lovely story your family is creating!

REVIEW PAGE

Dear Reader,

We hope this message finds you in good health and high spirits! We're reaching out because your opinion matters to us, and we'd love to hear what you think about "Family Health 2024."

If you've had the chance to dive into the book and explore its chapters, we would be incredibly grateful if you could take a moment to share your thoughts. Your review will not only provide valuable insights for us but also assist other readers in deciding if this book is the right fit for them.

Whether it's a few sentences or a detailed reflection, your feedback is instrumental in shaping the future of our work.

Thank you for being part of our journey towards healthier families. Your support means everything to us!

Warm regards,

Jocelyn J. Barker

Author, "Family Health 2024"

www.ingramcontent.com/pod-product-compliance
Lightning Source LLC
Chambersburg PA
CBHW070941260726
48661CB00003B/1076